LIVE WELL
EVERY DAY

DR ALEX GEORGE

LIVE WELL EVERY DAY

Your plan for a happy body and mind

aster

First published in Great Britain in 2021 by Aster,
an imprint of
Octopus Publishing Group Ltd
Carmelite House
50 Victoria Embankment
London EC4Y 0DZ
www.octopusbooks.co.uk

An Hachette UK Company
www.hachette.co.uk

Distributed in the US by
Hachette Book Group
1290 Avenue of the Americas
4th and 5th Floors
New York, NY 10104

Distributed in Canada by
Canadian Manda Group
664 Annette St
Toronto, Ontario, Canada M6S 2C8

ISBN 978-1-78325-431-6

A CIP catalogue record for this book is available from
the British Library.

Printed and bound in Italy

10 9 8 7 6 5 4 3 2 1

This FSC® label means that materials used for
the product have been responsibly sourced

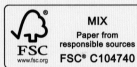

FSC
www.fsc.org

MIX
Paper from
responsible sources
FSC® C104740

Consultant Publisher Kate Adams
Deputy Art Director Jaz Bahra
Senior Editor Alex Stetter
Copy Editor Sarah Reece
Photographer Andrew Burton
Props Stylist Agathe Gits
Home Economist Lizzie Kamenetzky
Production Controller Allison Gonsalves

CONTENTS

INTRODUCTION

I first came up with the idea for *Live Well Every Day* about three years ago. I was thinking about the patients I was seeing in A&E and – accidents aside – how I could help them from reaching the point where they had to seek emergency help. If they looked at their health holistically and made small but consistent changes in the areas in which they were lacking, the cumulative effects would be enough not only to help them with their acute conditions, but also to have a profound effect on their health as a whole.

This idea had to go on the back burner for a while, as my life took a rather unexpected turn and I found myself in front of millions of TV viewers on a nightly basis – more of that later! But there's no doubt that in 2020 we all realized how much looking after our own physical and mental health matters. We had to stop and think about what we can do to live happier, healthier lives and to protect ourselves, as well as others.

My intention with this book is to put you back in the driving seat of your own health and wellbeing, and to show you how to take control and make incremental changes to your life that will last. *Live Well Every Day* is divided into seven chapters, named after what I believe are the fundamental areas of health. Not only are these pretty vital if we want to function at our best, they're also areas in which we can make changes and that's key. You can choose to have a positive effect on your health and happiness. I will talk to you about protecting your mental health, the power of good nutrition, the best sleep and relaxation techniques, and how important fitness is to both your physical and mental wellbeing. And I'll look at how having a purpose in life and a passion for living underpin everything.

I've always tried to be honest with you guys on my social media channels or whenever I appear on TV, and I've carried on with that here – even if it makes me cringe a bit in places! This book is a combination of my personal and professional experiences and I've included stories of the times when I've made mistakes or done things that haven't been healthy or helpful, and described how I addressed those things and turned my life around.

I hope this book will give you a personalized tool kit for a better you. Once you start to make changes, you won't look back, I promise.

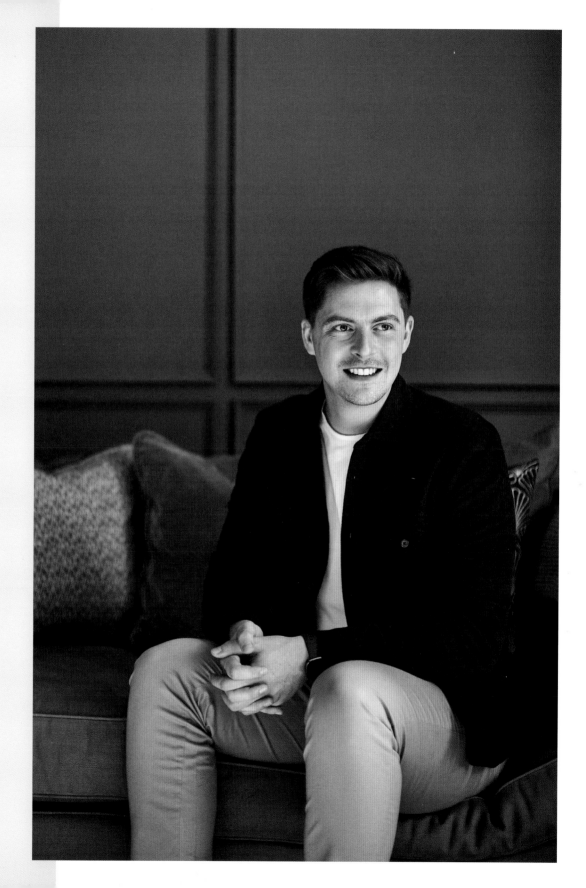

THIS BOOK IS
DEDICATED TO
LLŶR...

On 23 July 2020, I received the most devastating news imaginable: my beautiful little brother Llŷr had, unexpectedly, taken his own life. It came without warning and my family and I were in complete shock. We never thought it was possible to feel such pain; we simply couldn't believe it had happened.

Llŷr was only 19, with a career in medicine ahead of him. He already had a place at medical school and I was so, so proud of him. I miss him very much and, whatever I do, he is always in my thoughts.

Grief is an ongoing process, but I know I'll never get over losing my little brother. He and I often spoke about health, particularly mental health, and we were both passionate about ensuring children and young people are taught how to look after themselves when things go wrong.

Before Llŷr's death, I'd already been developing a 'mental health tool kit' with the aim of facilitating a structured curriculum for schools and universities around the country. This is something I intend to continue working on, to make sure children and young people who are struggling get the help they need. This work will now be carried out in memory of my little brother and will be a legacy for Llŷr.

Llŷr was very supportive about my ideas for this book and it's been very emotional writing it, as I wish he could see it being published. All I can do is dedicate this book to him – another legacy for Llŷr.

I am a positive person and I'm not going to let what has happened to my family change that. I still believe there is so much hope in the world. After Llŷr passed, someone very wise said to me, 'Life throws us into the deep end at times, but with the help of family and friends we can overcome even the most seemingly insurmountable challenges. Just know you're never alone.'

It's that last point that I want anyone reading this who is struggling to take onboard. If you feel you have no one to talk to, for whatever reason, there are fantastic charities out there, like Samaritans, Mind and CALM, and your GP as well, who *are* there for you, waiting to listen and ready to help (see Resources, page 233). If you are going through a tough time, please reach out. There is always hope of a better day.

1

YOUR HEALTH TODAY

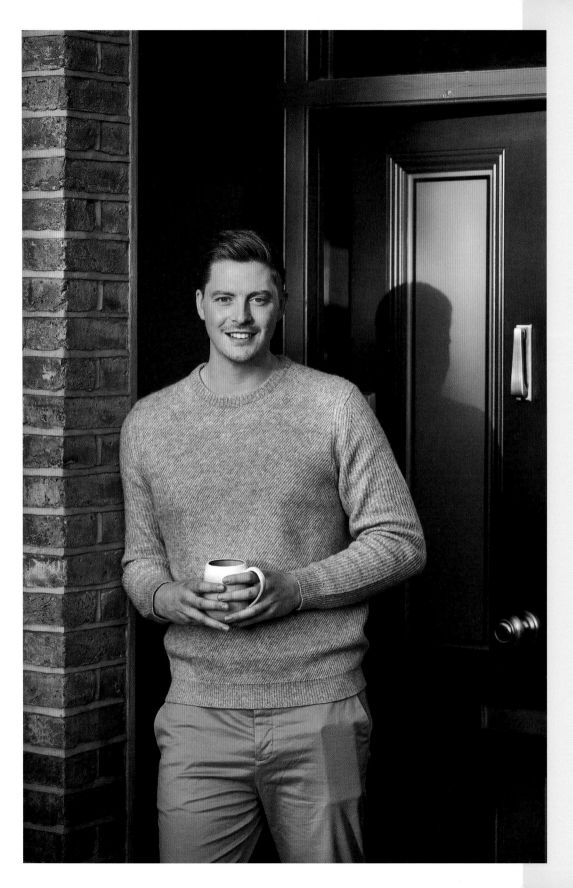

OUR RELATIONSHIP WITH OUR HEALTH

I've always been interested in how we can make small changes, whether in exercise or nutrition, in sleep or reducing stress. Little changes can accumulate and have a big impact on our overall health and happiness – an impact that is profound, but also sustainable. I'm not interested in fad diets and quick fixes; I'm talking about meaningful change that will improve our lives for good.

I know that most of us like to think we know what we should do in order to stay fit and healthy. In theory, if we eat well, exercise regularly, sleep for eight hours a night and keep an eye on our blood pressure, how hard can it be? In reality though, managing and maintaining our health can feel like an extreme juggling act at the best of times. Typically, we address health issues once they need a cure, rather than thinking about the possible preventative measures we might have taken to stay well. You could argue we expect too much from our bodies and only patch them up as and when needed, rather than monitoring their needs and stepping in before we reach crisis point. Sometimes that critical point is when you end up waiting in A&E to see me!

The truth is that the Covid-19 global pandemic tells a similar story, albeit on a larger scale. The crisis shone a much-needed light on what happens when we expect too much from an infrastructure like the NHS; we assumed it could run a metaphorical marathon without any training or fuel. As one of the thousands of NHS workers across the country who put their lives at risk to care for the most vulnerable, I saw what happens when a nation isn't ready for mass disease.

But that's the extreme end of the health spectrum. As an A&E doctor who is also part of the everyday health conversation, I am presented with similar individual unpreparedness all the time. Obviously there are a million reasons why people end up in A&E – and some of those reasons (especially accidents) have nothing to do with how well you look after yourself or how many times a week you exercise. But overall, I keep coming back to the same thing: if you do the right things to protect and take care of your body and mind, you give them the best chance of long-standing good health and avoiding visiting me in hospital.

THERE'S SO MUCH IN LIFE WE AREN'T IN CONTROL OF,
BUT DON'T FORGET THAT THERE IS A LOT THAT WE CAN
CONTROL TOO.

POSITIVE CHOICES

Everything you do has a direct impact on your day-to-day health, your immune system, your mental health, your metabolism, your bone density, your heart health, your blood pressure, your energy levels and how you fight disease generally. How and what you feed your mind and body, the choices you make every day, can affect how you tackle more severe medical problems should they come up – in conjunction with modern medicine, of course. Your lifestyle is often your body's biggest support system and the more robust you can make that, the more you can rely on it to get you through. Think of it as your life insurance policy.

I know, I know, it's easy for me to stand here in my scrubs and stethoscope and tell people what they should and shouldn't do. I don't want to patronize, but I do know from what patients, friends and family tell me that it can be hard to find the right information and make the best choices. So, I want this book to feel like the ultimate handbook to your health – a place you can find tips, facts and inspiration to replace some of your habits with healthier ones. I want to encourage you to think about how to keep your body and mind working effectively.

I am passionate about the fact that we all need to maintain our minds and bodies constantly and I want this book to help you feel you can take some control. I want you to feel equipped to make changes that are sustainable for life and help you prescribe the right things for your own body and mind. Because the truth is that the best thing I can do for you is to help you stay well, so you don't end up in my hospital waiting room.

Accidents aside, some of the people who end up in A&E are there because they have made potentially life-affecting bad choices in the past that end up culminating in illness. They have weakened their bodies and their minds to the point where it leads to bad health. A lot of people go through their lives eating badly, drinking to excess, smoking and not exercising, and they're fine until they hit 50 and then the wheels come off.

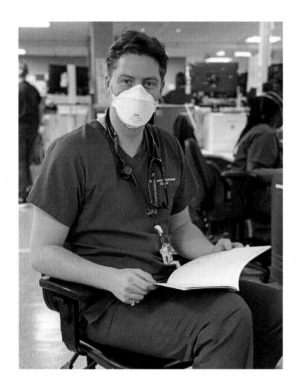
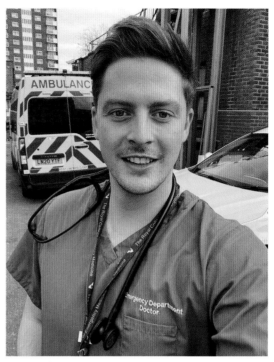
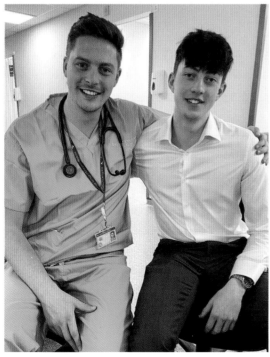
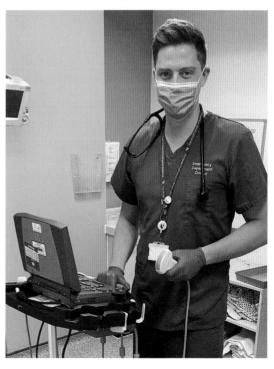

They get diabetes, they get high blood pressure, they get high cholesterol and then they have a massive heart attack. Now medicine can keep you alive for longer, but surely you'd want those later years to be ones you can enjoy, not ones spent having to deal with a multitude of health issues. Issues that you could potentially have avoided if you had been just a bit more sensible when you were younger.

We're lucky enough to be living through a time when life expectancy is longer than ever. While smoking rates may be decreasing, Type 2 diabetes, obesity, dementia and mental health issues are on the rise. There is an increasing awareness of the importance of being healthy when we're younger and building a strong foundation to ensure our good health is retained in our later years. It may not always be what many people want to hear, but we need to look after our bodies when we're young to ensure it lasts us into old age.

CASE STUDY – GEOFF

I saw a gentleman the other day, let's call him Geoff. A big strapping man and really strong, although advancing in years. He told me he had always been an athlete and played a lot of sport and had physical jobs. He'd always been very health conscious, eaten well and, since retiring, walks everywhere and lifts weights every day. His muscles were strong, he wasn't frail and his skeletal strength was amazing. He just looked healthy and alert, with bright eyes and colour in his cheeks. He honestly looked like a man 20 years younger. And it was only now, well past retirement age, that he had to come in to see a doctor about a few health problems. Geoff was really impressive.

The simple reason for all this is the way he looked after himself. And it struck me that he had made the right choices in his life; he respected his body and knew that if he looked after it, fortune willing, it would last him a long time. And he was right. I think we should all be more like Geoff.

MEDICINE AND ME

In all honesty the last few years do all feel like a bit of blur really. Thinking back to summer 2018 when this all started, I had a life-changing decision to make: carry on as a doctor in A&E or enter the *Love Island* villa as a contestant. I was originally approached via Instagram and asked to take part in the show – I genuinely thought it was a joke at first! I was offered an interview, but I kept saying no. It's funny now when I think about it – I was probably the only contestant on the show who wasn't even sure I wanted to be there, or wanted what was to come afterwards. One thing I would say is that being a reality TV star was never part of my plan or ambition, but I feel very lucky it provided the platform for everything I am doing now.

In my role as a doctor, the patients are the key to everything – I love hearing their stories, finding out about their lives and learning from them. I always tell medical students to make sure they learn something new from every patient they meet, no matter how irrelevant it may seem. People are genuinely amazing and I hope I never lose that sense of wonder about humans. As a doctor you have the privilege of being there to witness someone's best and worst moments, with the opportunity to help and make a difference, and the privilege of that never stops blowing my mind.

Post-*Love Island*, I'm now in a position to reach out to my large audience and share my knowledge and experience, to give something back to all those patients I've admired and who told me their stories, and to educate everyone about the part they can play in their own health, highlighting the things they can control, with the aim that this will genuinely mean fewer visits to GPs and hospitals for all. I really want this book to help tackle health issues that affect everyone, especially millennials, who I believe can make a huge change to their own health outlook if they understand the basic principles of long-lasting health.

The first and most important principle is that our mental health is at the core of everything. I don't think it is an exaggeration to say that every part of our body in some way affects every other part and our mental health is no different. How we feel and the health of our mental space are the key to everything else working as it should. It affects what and how we eat, how we move, how we sleep and how we manage stress. Everything pivots around mental wellness, something I found out first-hand during my medical training (see page 50).

HOW IS YOUR HEALTH TODAY?

While I may be a doctor and this book may be packed with practical health advice, I must also say that it's no substitute for a visit to your doctor when needs must (see Chapter 7 for more information). But something I'd encourage you to do now is to take a blank piece of paper and a pen. Then just write down whatever comes to mind about how your health is today. Scribble notes if that's easier than writing full sentences; no one else needs to read it. You can even use voice notes if you like. I just want to get you thinking about health conditions you might be struggling with or have not yet addressed. How you feel on a daily basis, how you think your diet is, whether you feel fit, energetic, strong, happy…

This is just a starting point, food for thought. It's a useful exercise though for placing yourself in the present – don't think about the person you used to be at high school or who you want to be in the future. Take a health inventory of where you are right now.

DR GOOGLE WILL SEE YOU NOW…

One reason people end up in A&E is fear. There are a lot of statistics about people (particularly men) ignoring symptoms and not seeking professional medical advice when needed, leaving their conditions until they're critical and they have no choice but to seek emergency treatment. And it's this fear, the fear of finally knowing, that brings them to my door. To be fair, I think the medical world has to shoulder some of the blame for this – we could have been better at disseminating medical information in the past. We've tried to own medical information, rather than sharing it and therefore empowering people.

It's common for people to google their symptoms, get a worst-case scenario – a totally non-professional diagnosis – and then hide away worrying about it. There's no medical resource online or elsewhere that gives the other side of the story: how a healthy lifestyle has long-term benefits when it comes to developing certain conditions, allowing you to be better able to deal with them should they come along, with an improved likelihood of recovery.

I WANT TO GIVE PEOPLE MORE INFORMATION SO THEY CAN SEE THE BENEFITS OF A HEALTHY LIFESTYLE FROM THE GET-GO AND MAKE THE RIGHT CHOICES AS THEY PROGRESS THROUGH LIFE.

A QUICK HEALTH MOT

Forgive the car analogy (once a pistonhead…), but, just as you keep your vehicle roadworthy with a yearly MOT, so it's useful to do the same for your body. I also think it's important to know your baseline health before you start making any changes – otherwise how will you know what's working and what isn't?

When a patient is in A&E we'll check and record their 'vitals' and it's amazing how little these numbers mean to many people. They have no idea what their blood pressure should be, let alone what it is.

So I'd urge you to record the measurements listed on the next page, if you know them, and try to find them out if you don't.

I can't diagnose through these pages and I don't try to. Instead, what I'm trying to let you know is that there is so much you can do, every day, to boost your all-round health and live your best life. And by keeping tabs on what's normal for you, you can quickly recognize what's not – and take action.

♥

YOUR HEALTH MOT

Maintaining a healthy weight – neither under- nor overweight for your height and frame – is undeniably important. Forget appearance, it's about how your body works. I'm no advocate of standing on the scales every day, but it's a good idea to do so from time to time, so you know what a healthy weight looks and feels like for you and can take action if it's heading in the wrong direction.

Body mass index (BMI), while not without its critics, is a useful measurement to know what the healthy weight zones are for a person of your age, gender and height. More on this on page 110.

Waist measurement is another useful one to be aware of. A measurement of greater than 80cm (31½in) for women, 94cm (37in) for most men, or 90cm (35in) for South Asian men is a risk factor for Type 2 diabetes.

Resting heart rate (RHR) is the number of times per minute your heart beats while at rest. This number gives a snapshot of how well your heart muscle is working, and it's also a good metric for fitness (lower RHR can equal better cardio fitness).

Blood pressure is a measure of the force your body uses to pump blood around your circulatory system. It's given as two figures and measured in millimetres of mercury. Healthy blood pressure is generally considered to be around 120/80mmHg. Low blood pressure, which can make you prone to dizziness and fainting, can be caused by some medications or may indicate dehydration or heart problems. High blood pressure tends to be a result of smoking, drinking to excess, not exercising or being overweight. It's a risk factor for coronary heart disease and kidney disease.

Having too much of a fatty substance called cholesterol in your blood can block blood vessels, leading to a heart attack or stroke. High cholesterol can be hereditary but is more often a result of poor diet and lifestyle choices. We measure it via a blood test and look at various different markers. Ones for you to be aware of are total cholesterol (good and bad, this should be 5 or below) and LDL (the bad type, which should be 3 or below).

YOUR VITALS

Your weight

....

Your body mass index (see page 110)

....

Your waist measurement

....

Your resting heart rate

....

Your blood pressure

....

Your total cholesterol and your LDL (bad) cholesterol

....

LOOK INTO YOUR FUTURE

Your family health history is also important. While many diseases are caused by our modern lifestyles, there are many others with a genetic component. Finding out if any of your family have certain conditions can help you protect yourself and be attuned to any early signs in your own body. So be a family health detective and ask your loved ones the following seven questions:

- **Have any of my close relatives had cancer – what type and at what age?**
- **Has anyone in the family had cardiovascular disease, including high blood pressure or a stroke?**
- **Is there a history of high cholesterol?**
- **Is there a history of depression or other mental health conditions?**
- **Are there any other major diseases in the family?**
- **What did my grandparents and great-grandparents die of?**
- **Has anyone experienced fertility issues or early menopause?**

I'm well aware this sounds like a pretty downbeat conversation to be having with your folks. But hey, it could well have its upsides too. You might find out you come from a long line of centenarians! My point is, it's empowering to find out as much as you can about the hand you've been dealt when it comes to your health. And that's because there's always something you can do to prevent potential issues or improve your odds. Think of it like future-proofing. Knowledge is power.

How's your diary looking?

When was your last eye test, dental appointment, cervical smear, flu vaccination? You're not sure? I don't blame you, it's hard to keep track. But it's really important to keep up to date with appointments and not put off routine screening or vaccination when they're offered. Trust me, nothing is given out for free in health care unless we know it works!

Turn to page 223 to record your last appointments and when your next ones are due.

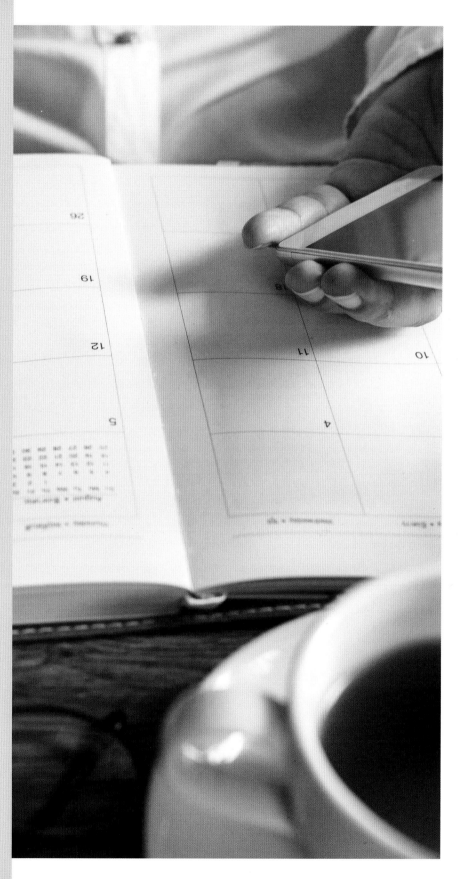

HOW TO USE THIS BOOK

I want *Live Well Every Day* to be both a health transformation plan for you to follow and an everyday reference guide to good health and wellbeing. I've poured my heart and soul into these pages and, as I do on social media, I've been happy to share a lot of my own experiences. I figure it helps to know that whatever you're going through, someone's been there before you. There's lots you can pick up from how other people dealt with something (or not, as is often the case).

Over my years as a med student, junior doctor and in A&E, I've seen thousands of different health conditions. So I bring some of that insight into this book too, in the form of stories and case studies. I think it all helps to bring the information I'm trying to convey to life.

By all means use the index (see page 235) to look up particular issues and find my advice. Or perhaps you'll read a chapter that jumps out at you first. In the next section, you'll see that I've broadly divided my writing into seven chapters, representing the seven ways of health that I think are key for our all-round physical and mental health. They are:

1. Passion & Purpose

2. A Healthy Mind

3. Nutrition

4. Fitness & Flexibility

5. Recharge

6. Sex & Relationships

7. Taking Control of Your Health

If one or more of these elements is out of kilter, your overall wellbeing is likely to suffer. But these seven ways of health are also interlinked and this may not be immediately obvious. If you're sleeping badly, for example, your nutrition the next day may suffer because you're tired and make poor food choices. And if you're living a sedentary life and not getting any exercise or fresh air, your sleep is going to be impacted. You don't have to be perfect in each of these seven areas; I'm sure there will be some that immediately stand out to you as needing more attention than others. But what I'm suggesting is you try and achieve a balance across all seven. They really will all help each other out.

For those of you who are already keen to make some positive changes to your health and your life, I've designed each chapter to be super practical, with lots of self-assessments, takeaway advice and actionable points. At the end of every chapter you'll find a weekly challenge, where I suggest one change or a choice of changes you can try to keep up over the course of seven days and notice the difference. I know life is busy and stressful and big changes can sometimes feel overwhelming, so I've also included some mini actions you can take – 'What can you do TODAY?' I added those to show that, sometimes, even the tiniest change is all you need to feel you've achieved something. And that, in turn, starts you on a course to lasting positive behaviour change. I've seen it in patients – and I've tried it for myself.

In the last section of the book (see page 220), I've included various worksheets, activities and pages for your notes, so you can keep tabs on how you're doing. Plus there are lists of trusted resources (see page 233), for when you need more help.

I really hope you find this book useful and empowering and that it becomes something you share with friends and family, and return to yourself again and again. It's been an honour and a privilege to write it, and I hope it helps you live well, every day.

2

THE SEVEN WAYS OF HEALTH

1

WHEN YOU FEEL FULFILLED, THE TOUGH SIDES OF LIFE ARE EASIER TO BEAR. IT'S NEVER TOO LATE TO FIND YOUR PURPOSE: PURSUE YOUR PASSIONS AND GET ON THE RIGHT TRACK.

PASSION & PURPOSE

I try not to make a habit of quoting famous German philosophers, but I came across this and I'd like to share it with you: 'He who has a why to live for can bear almost any how.' That's by Friedrich Nietzsche and, without wanting to appear too highbrow, I think it sums up this chapter pretty well.

Everyone needs a purpose; it's what gets us out of bed in the morning, drives and energizes us, and gives us a feeling of belonging and a sense of fulfilment. And the opposite can be true of not having a purpose. Living a life without purpose can result in anxiety, depression and low self-esteem. It can also be behind any poor lifestyle choices we make, such as bad diet, drinking too much alcohol or other potentially harmful vices. By using these things to compensate for lack of meaning, we're in danger of our lives spiralling out of control.

I was lucky: I knew what I wanted to do from a young age and have managed to follow my passion and turn it into a career with purpose. I was fortunate that I had the support to do this and I'm grateful for that every day.

Finding what your purpose is has no age limit. Life being what it is, not many people have the opportunity to stop and take stock of where they are and whether they're fulfilling their true purpose. Bills need to be paid and kids need to be raised, I totally get that. But the flip side of that is, if you do invest a little time into thinking about what makes you happy, and if there's some way of combining that with the talents you already have and the values you hold, then the benefits will directly impact your daily life. Without getting too spiritual, I truly believe that finding your purpose and pursuing it is one of the most fundamental things you can do to achieve a fulfilled and balanced life. So it's worth taking the time to do so – doctor's orders!

I want to use this chapter to help people do just that; to look at where they are in their lives and to ask themselves if they feel truly fulfilled and, if not, what can they do about it. I'm going to tell you how I found my purpose and what it took to pursue that to get to where I am today. I'll then share with you tools to help you work out what your true passions are and where your ultimate purpose lies. If you think you've lost your way or are not fulfilled in life, you can assess your path and then make adjustments that set you back on track. Even if you are content and feel that you're on the right path already, it's also worth taking stock – if nothing else it will confirm that you're doing what you've always wanted to do and that you're on the right track.

CHOOSING HAPPINESS

I'm going to start by telling you about one of the most inspirational patients I've ever met. It's not a happy story, but it illustrates what I'm going to be talking about in this chapter.

Let's call her Anna. She was born in Eastern Europe, came to the UK as a child and ended up in a foster home. She had a terrible time and left as soon as she could, still in her teenage years. Anna loved children, but an early diagnosis of cancer and the treatment for it left her unable to have her own, so she chose a career in education so she could at least work with them. She adored her work and told me she could relate to difficult children because her upbringing was so troubled; she was taking her negative experience and turning it into a positive one.

Unhappily, Anna's cancer returned and when I met her she didn't have long to live. But when she told me her story she was laughing and smiling. Initially I couldn't understand how someone who had struggled so much could be so upbeat, but she said, 'Alex, what other option is there? If these are my last days then I'd rather spend them being happy.'

Anna was so inspiring; despite terrible setbacks, she had pursued her passion and made it her purpose. She was fulfilled and, importantly, she chose to be happy. Sadly, I sometimes see people who are the opposite of Anna. I remember one middle-aged high-flying businessman who had been boozing since his early 20s and was in A&E with severe alcoholic liver disease. He told me he was rich but miserable, turning to vodka to numb the emptiness he felt. It seemed to me that he had found his passion – accumulating money – but not his purpose.

A lack of purpose can result in us making bad choices and ultimately harming ourselves. There's nothing quite like earning a living from doing something you love, but making money purely for the sake of it rarely leads to true fulfilment and happiness. There were alternative careers open to me that could have been more lucrative than working for the NHS, but I followed my passion, found my purpose and my success followed on from that.

In my experience, living your life with a sense of purpose gives you the confidence to seek new opportunities. *Love Island* is a good example of that. Trying something new doesn't always work out, however, and I've experienced some failures alongside the success – some might say *Love Island* is a good example of that too! I've learned to roll with the punches though and that becomes easier if you're doing something you feel you were born to do.

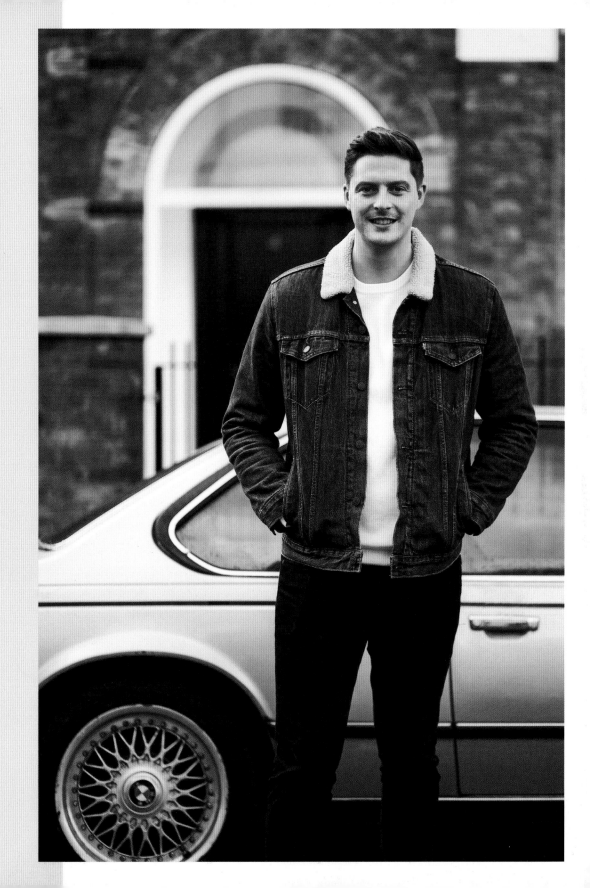

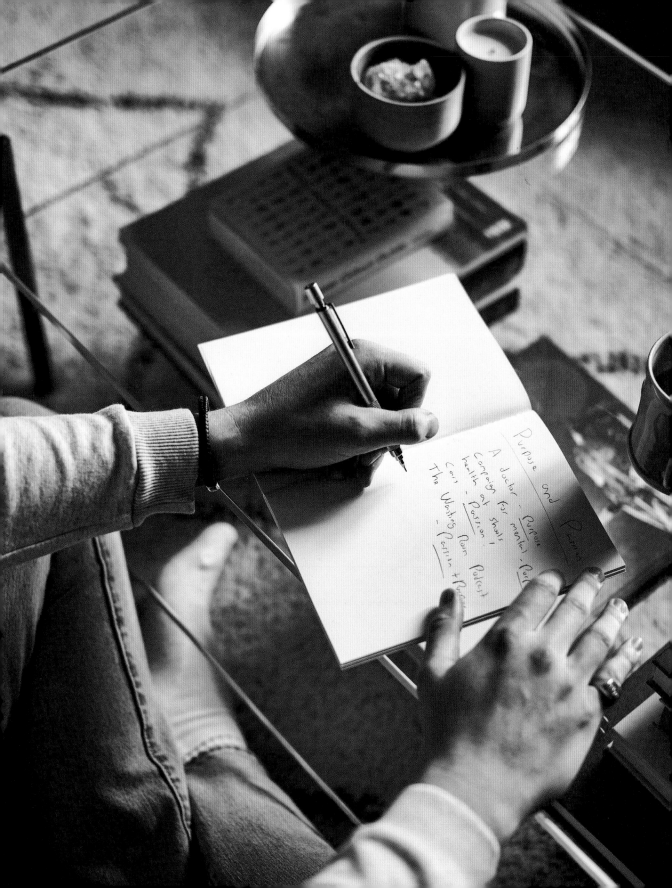

THE PURPOSE PRESCRIPTION

There's a school of thought that says purpose sits at the intersection of talent, values, passion and expertise. Well, that was definitely the case for me and, even though I wasn't consciously making the connection, my talents, values and passions, plus the expertise I accumulated by following them, gave me my purpose: to be a doctor and to help people.

Going back to the beginning though, I'd say my real talent was my emotional intelligence. If you were to ask my parents what I was like when I was younger, they would tell you – once they'd got the embarrassing stories out of the way – that I was always in tune with other people and that I could get a good grasp of what someone was like after being with them for just a short time. As far back as I can remember, I've always been interested in other people and it's been a real asset, not just at work, but in my everyday life too.

My passions are a bit random, as on the face of it they're poles apart. First was my love of science: physics, chemistry, biology, you name it, if it involved putting on a lab coat I was into it. At the other end of the spectrum was my need for a bit of excitement – whether on the rugby pitch or tennis court, or later on in very fast cars. I do like a bit of adrenaline!

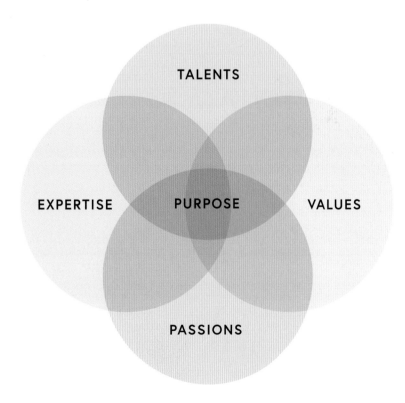

I HAVE FOUND THAT IN LIFE, POSITIVITY AND PURPOSE GO HAND-IN-HAND.

My values come from my parents. My mum is one of the most caring people I know, always doing her utmost to help others. She used to say to me, you can do anything in life as long as you put your mind to it. She's also a stickler for rules and making sure things were done for the right reasons. My dad was a policeman, so doing the wrong thing was never an option with him either! Between them they instilled in me a deep sense of right and wrong, which I carry with me today.

So, a naturally intuitive and empathetic adrenaline junkie with a passion for science and biology and a desire to help people – my path seems pretty obvious when you look at it like that, right?! Just to top it off, I used to love watching A&E hospital shows on TV – they gave me a real buzz and I used to imagine myself as the doctor attending an accident and dealing with the bleeding and drama. It was meant to be!

REDEFINE FAILURE

While I may have found my purpose at an early age, the route to becoming an A&E doctor wasn't an easy one. It's an old adage, I know, but I really believe that you learn more from your failures than from your successes. I didn't have an easy time at school; I was quite bright, but I had undiagnosed dyslexia (I was only formally diagnosed after medical school) and I struggled with traditional learning and had a very short attention span. I always try to find a positive though and, if I look at my life now, my ability to juggle lots of different things at the same time probably comes from not being able to focus on any one thing for too long.

In addition to the issues mentioned above, when I went to secondary school I was badly bullied. This was a time when my sensitivity set me apart for different reasons – it was tough and my results suffered. The reason I'm sharing this with you guys is because I want to demonstrate that, despite being lucky enough to know what my purpose in life was, there were still many barriers in the way. Hopefully you'll read this and see that there are ways of overcoming such obstacles and that tenacity is an important factor in following your passion. I turned a corner at school when I decided I wasn't going to stand for the bullying anymore. I got together with my friends and we sorted it out by showing the bullies they were dealing with a group of us and not one person on their own. Bullies tend not to like it when the odds are evened out a bit. From there my confidence grew, as did my popularity; I started to do well at sport, my schoolwork improved and I left school on a high. And I learned many lessons from the experience of being bullied, particularly when it came to empathy.

Unfortunately, however, the rest of my journey to med school wasn't plain sailing either. I'd done my work experience at Morriston Hospital in Swansea and loved my time there. I'd also got my place at the University of Liverpool School of Medicine lined up. I was so excited! When I got my A-level results, I'd missed out on my chemistry pass by two marks. Despite my head teacher calling the med school to give me a reference, they wouldn't budge. It was a big setback, but I dusted myself off, redid the coursework and applied to Peninsula Medical School at the University of Plymouth, with success this time. I remember thinking to myself, don't forget the taste of this, because it was so bitter, and never let it happen again.

I took the fire that failure had lit inside me to med school and, when I left five years later, it was with a distinction and in the top one per cent in the country. Job done.

Empathy is one of the most important abilities we can develop – in learning how to share another person's feelings and emotions, and putting ourselves in their shoes to understand a situation more fully, we learn more about our own emotions too.

'LIVE YOUR LIFE!'

Talking of inspiration, I'd like to mention here my very close friend Freya Barlow. We met at med school and I would definitely have always put her forward as somebody who had found a way to combine their passion with their purpose. She had the kindest heart and the most empathy of anyone I've ever met. She was the purest person and, even though she studied hard, she still managed to find time to raise money for several charities.

Just before we were due to take our exams, she was diagnosed with advanced leukaemia and had to start chemo treatment immediately. Despite having to have a bone marrow transplant, she still sat her exams and even ran a marathon a few months later to raise money for one of her charities. She was such an inspiration.

Sadly the treatment wasn't successful and she was given two to three weeks to live. Before she went home for the last time, we threw a big ball at the university in her honour. The last time I saw her she said to me, 'Say yes to everything and live a life worth remembering.'

So when I'm confronted with problems or offered opportunities I always think, what would Freya say? She was in the forefront of my mind when I was asked to go on *Love Island*. While I was worrying about whether a doctor should go on a reality TV show and how would it affect my career, I could hear Freya's voice saying, 'Go for it, live your life!' She would have loved me being on the show – she would have laughed her head off!

Now I tend to throw myself into things, whether I feel comfortable doing them or not. My rationale is that, if I'm following my purpose, then all these opportunities are part of the same journey. Freya would have made the best doctor, but she didn't get the chance, so if something intimidates me or if I'm having a hard time of it, I always bring it back to her and never take things for granted.

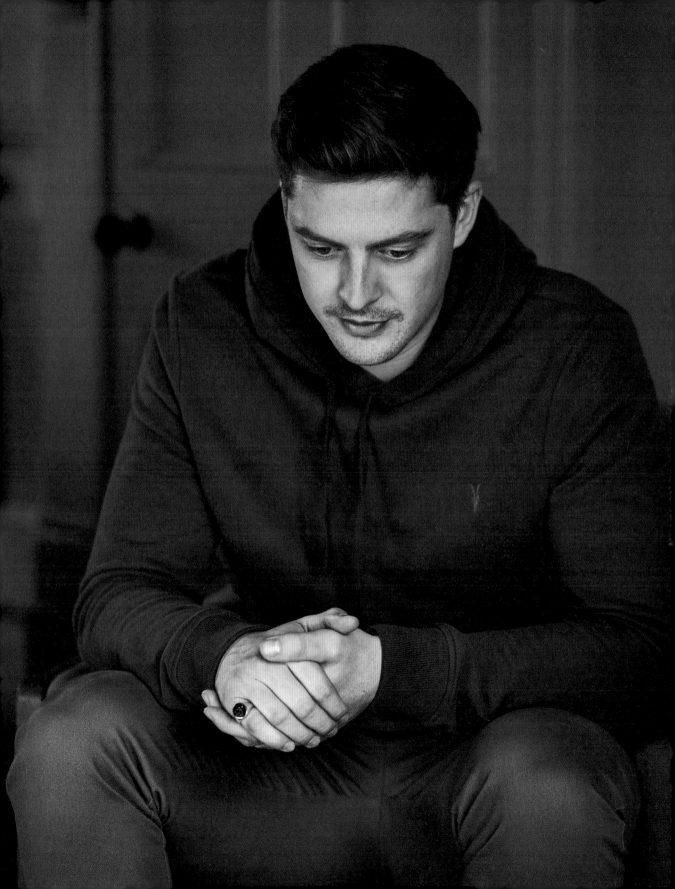

IN MY EXPERIENCE, LIVING YOUR LIFE WITH A SENSE
OF PURPOSE GIVES YOU THE CONFIDENCE TO START
SEEKING OUT AND TRYING NEW OPPORTUNITIES.

THE POWER OF PURPOSE

When I came off *Love Island* I felt like I'd lost myself. In many ways it had been an interesting experience, but deep down I felt I'd been distracted from what I should have been doing and wasn't following my purpose. As soon as I went back to A&E, everything clicked back into place and after a while I began to see the benefits of being on a show like *Love Island*. First of all, my appearance on the show gave my social media following a massive boost – my Instagram followers alone went from 268 to over a million (it's currently nearly 2 million) and I now have 100,000 subscribers on YouTube. An incredible platform! I thought long and hard about what content to share with my followers and initially I simply let people into my life and shared an insight into my A&E experiences.

But when the Covid-19 pandemic hit in early 2020, I realized I could do my bit and help get important public health messages out via my channels. I created content that gave advice about handwashing, mental health and how best to protect yourself from Covid-19, and those videos were watched and shared millions of times. It was then I understood that, rather than detracting from my role as a doctor, *Love Island* had enabled me to fulfil my purpose further. It gave me the opportunity to connect with people – people who may have missed important medical information otherwise – and help them negotiate the pandemic. When that happened, I got a real sense of what I talked about earlier, of living a life with a sense of purpose and how that gives you the confidence to start seeking out new opportunities. An elderly patient once told me that the things he regretted the most were the things he didn't do, not the ones he did. My purpose was helped by going on the show and, looking, back I couldn't be prouder for taking that risk.

FIND YOUR 'WHY', THEN FIGURE OUT YOUR 'HOW'

Whether we know it or not, we're all looking for fulfilment. When we satisfy that need, it makes the difficulties and downsides of life easier to bear. I find that even if I have a terrible day in A&E, I can deal with it, because in some way I've contributed to the health and betterment of my patients. That is my purpose, my reason for being, and knowing that I'm doing what I was born to do predisposes me to deal with anything life wants to throw at me.

Remember the Nietzsche quote I started the chapter with? 'He who has a why to live for can bear almost any how.' Another person who was fond of quoting that was Viktor Frankl, an Austrian Holocaust survivor, neurologist, psychiatrist and author. Frankl, who like millions of Jewish people suffered terribly during the Second World War, found that meaning and purpose were especially important in situations of extreme misery. He found that his fellow inmates who maintained a sense of purpose while incarcerated managed to find ways to survive and lived longer than those who didn't.

For Frankl, finding one's purpose was literally a matter of life and death.

MY BIG SECRET

One thing I had to overcome in following my purpose was my squeamishness at the sight of blood! I also used to faint at the sight of a needle – not great for a wannabe doctor! However, I knew it was not an insurmountable challenge, so all I did was expose myself to what I was afraid of. My first ever work experience day was in orthopedic surgery watching a knee replacement and I was just swaying! Luckily someone got hold of me and sat me in the corner and I was fine.

I've seen everything now – legs hanging off, hands missing – but I still don't like eyeballs hanging out. Apart from that, I can pretty much handle anything; this yet again shows that if you find your true purpose, nothing will keep you from it – even fainting on the job!

VISUALIZE YOUR PURPOSE

When it comes to passion and purpose, seeing really is believing. Starting a mood board can be a great help in working out what it is you really want from life. To-do lists have their place, but they normally come with a deadline and therefore add pressure. By slowly building up a pictorial version of what you like and where you want to be, you'll not only be actively taking a step towards fulfilment every time you add to it, but it will be something you can look at and contemplate whenever you have a spare couple of minutes. Much better than looking at a boring old list!

Now you know I'm all about the socials, and there are plenty of apps you could utilize to do this, but in this instance I think creating something physical has the greatest impact. You could use a sheet of card, a corkboard, the door of your fridge or even a wall that could maybe do with brightening up. Whatever you choose, start by putting a favourite photo of yourself in the centre, then start to add images, quotes, photographs, clippings from newspapers and magazines, whatever you can lay your hands on that relates to your passions and where you see fulfilment. Don't overthink it or try and 'curate' it – if something speaks to you, stick it up there.

And don't worry about 'finishing' it – your mood board can be, and should be, an ever-evolving thing. If you're reluctant to let other people see it, then that's fine, just make sure you put it somewhere that *you* will see it every day, so that the images get a chance to speak to your subconscious mind, giving you a focus for the day and encouraging you another step closer to fulfilment.

The science of visualization

Looking at your mood board is a form of visualization – a method used by successful people the world over, from elite athletes to business leaders. But I think it comes into its own as a tool for personal contentment. Brain studies have revealed that thinking can activate the same pathways in the brain as doing, so when you visualize something, you're practising for the real thing. Visualization is a proven tool for motivation, improved self-confidence and self-efficacy, reduced stress and anxiety. Combine it with intentions or affirmations, spoken out loud. In short? Every time you look at or call to mind an element of your mood board, you're one step closer to realizing it.

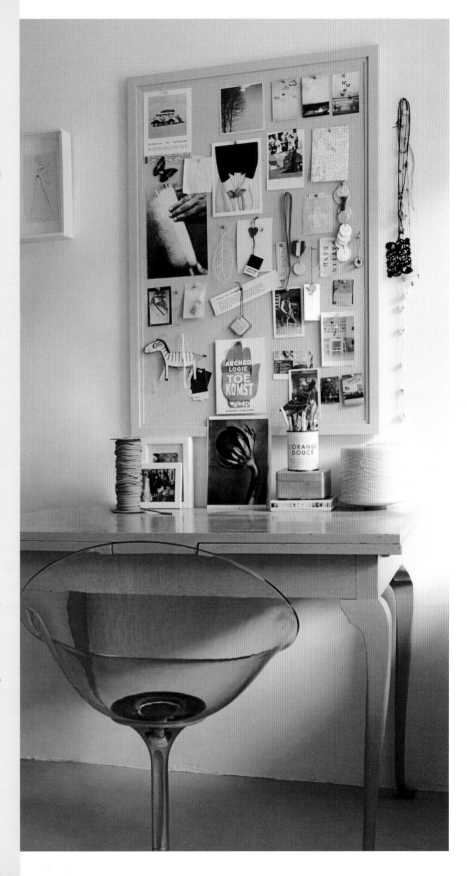

FIND YOUR PURPOSE

How do you find your purpose? Here, I've put together seven questions to help you identify your passions, talents, values and skills, from which you can identify your purpose (or purposes – yes, you can have more than one).

Be open-minded when answering these questions. Most importantly, be honest. Think about what's important to you, not what your parents' ambitions were for you or where your position in life dictates you should be. What do *you* want? What are you passionate about? What makes you tick?

Put your answers for each question in order of importance, then give each answer a score from 1–5 depending on how close you are to achieving or fulfilling them (with 1 being 'not very close' and 5 being 'just about there'). Take a look at those scores. Are you content with how close you are to achieving those things? If so, great. If not, then those should move to the top of your list.

1. **What gets you up in the morning?**

2. **What makes you come alive?**

3. **What are your strengths?**

4. **Where in your life do you think you are at your most useful?**

5. **What were you passionate about as a child?**

6. **What's your idea of success?**

7. **What is on your bucket list?**

Once you've identified what's important to you, think of ways that you can align your goals with how you already spend your time. For example, if it's work that gets you up in the morning but you wish it was something else, consider how you can integrate more of what was important to you as a kid into your life or career now. If the thought of being a good parent makes you come alive, look at how you can incorporate other things on your list into bringing up your kids.

Look at your answers and think about how you can pursue them. Perhaps a change of career is in order, or a change of social habits or hobbies. Don't discount anything; it's normal to have several different purposes and they can change over time.

Having identified your purpose, you can do something every day that is aligned with it and brings you closer to fulfilling it. Even something as simple as setting an intention every day is a step in the right direction.

SAY IT OUT LOUD!

Make an intention for the day, every day. Before you even get out of bed, identify one thing you'll do that day, no matter how small, that you'll stick to. Say it out loud to give intention to your purpose for that day. Don't be shy; you may be new to self-talk, but you'll soon get used to it. I do it every day as I walk to work – I don't even notice the funny looks any more!

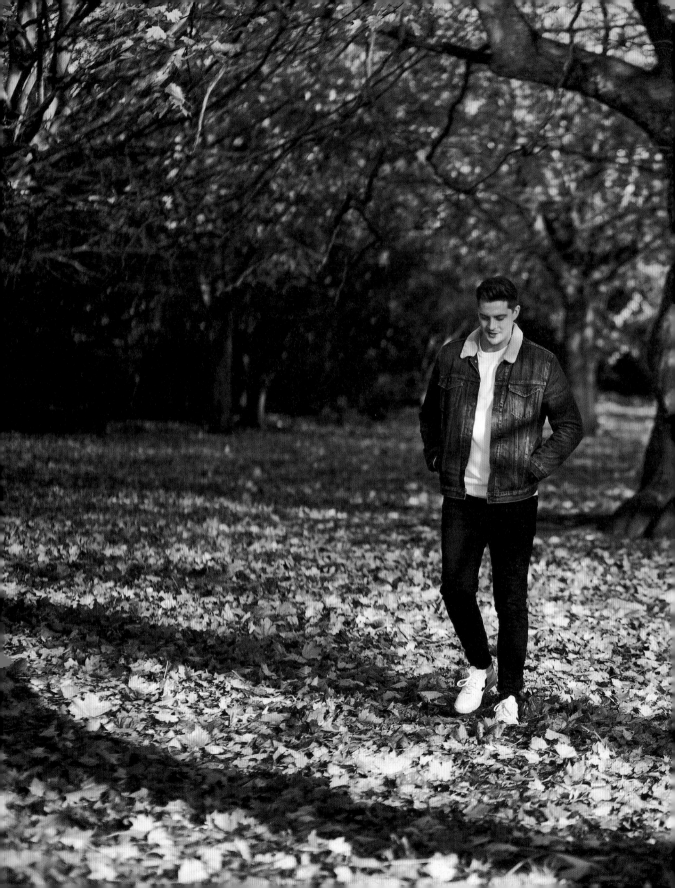

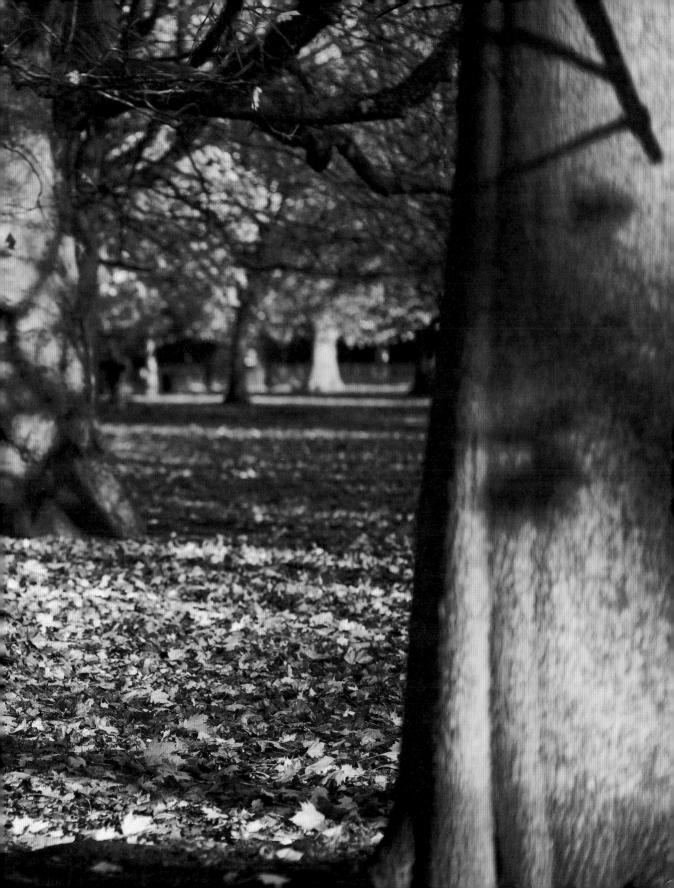

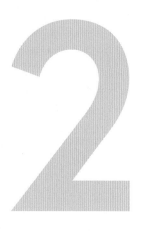

MENTAL AND PHYSICAL
HEALTH GO TOGETHER:
INVESTING TIME AND
ENERGY IN YOUR ROUTINE,
EXERCISE, DIET, SLEEP AND
RELATIONSHIPS IS GOOD
FOR MIND AND BODY.

A HEALTHY MIND

For me, mental and physical health cannot be separated. Put simply, if you can't do the things you enjoy in life because you are physically restricted by some illness or ailment, your mental health suffers. If you have poor mental health and don't keep up with your hobbies, exercise or healthy diet, then your physical health suffers. Looking after both your body and mind will ultimately lead to a happier and healthier you.

Something I have noticed since I qualified as a doctor is how many patients come to hospital with a physical symptom, but it turns out that mental difficulties are at the root of the problem. Take heart palpitations, for example: the condition is an awareness of your own heartbeat and there are a number of causes, some serious and some benign (see page 217). On many occasions I have seen terrified young patients with a racing pulse come to A&E because they believe they are having a heart attack. However, once I have assessed them fully and ruled out any serious cause, we often find out there is a very different issue at the root of the problem. Anxiety attacks can have very real physical symptoms, and a person experiencing one may attribute these to an underlying physical illness. When I dig deeper into the background of the patient, it can turn out they are under a huge amount of stress and strain, often with a trigger leading to a panic attack. It is a stark reminder to me of how interlinked our physical and mental health really are.

Unfortunately there's a stigma attached to the phrase 'mental health', which can be damaging in terms of perception and can also stop people from asking for help if they're struggling. When we talk about 'physical health', we think of fitness, exercise and positivity, but for some reason the words 'mental health' only have negative connotations. Think about it, have you ever heard someone say, 'So-and-so has really great mental health'? No, me neither.

So, I want to change the conversation and take a positive approach to discussing mental health. This chapter is about how to achieve a happy and healthy mind, one that complements your physical health. The Fitness & Flexibility chapter in this book looks at ways to improve your physical health and, in doing so, helps you navigate certain illnesses and conditions. And that's what I want this chapter to do too, but for your mental health: it's about focus, having a positive mindset and being able to deal with things should life suddenly throw you a curveball.

What's good for your body really is good for your mind and vice versa. Your health and happiness shouldn't be compartmentalized but treated as a whole, a state of being that is the sum of both, a 360-degree approach. And how happy you are and how well you feel are the summation of all these elements of your life.

MY EXPERIENCE: ANXIETY ISLAND

Love Island was obviously massive for me and I'll always be grateful for the platform it gave me. Yet despite it being a positive thing to do in many ways, it doesn't define me – how I dealt with being on the show does.

Newton's Law dictates that 'every action has an equal and opposite reaction' and I believe that is true in *all* aspects of life – you can't have a positive without a negative. For me this was most apparent with fame, which brought incredible opportunities, but was a burden too. The first six months after leaving the show felt like a complete blur. When I look back, I am not actually sure it was 'me' experiencing it. It's hard to describe what it's like to re-enter a world that has been watching your every move for weeks, where every conversation you had on screen became tabloid fodder. To have provided that entertainment, but also to know that I couldn't remember half of what was said, messed with my mind. The first time I turned on my phone and saw that over one million complete strangers were following me on Instagram, looking for me to update them on my life, was quite a moment.

Basically, I didn't understand how my new reality worked; I found myself saying, 'What the hell is this?!' at least once a day. I look back now and realize it was a total mental whirlwind – it's impossible to describe the headspace – especially as it seems odd to admit you are struggling with fame having just been on arguably the most talked-about reality TV show in modern times. That's the very reason people go on the show!

I soon recognized that big life changes – even positive ones – can really rock you, so I decided to get some therapy to help navigate this new world. I also spoke to the show's producers and, based on my experience, confirmed the importance of all contestants being offered counselling once they leave the island to help them readjust to life outside the bubble. It's a duty of care the show has taken very seriously.

My post-*Love Island* situation is obviously not an everyday one, but going back to Newton's theory, any major change in someone's life, whether that be moving to a new town, getting a new job or receiving a promotion, has the potential to create mental-wellness issues. Don't feel bad if the good things that happen to you also bring a level of anxiety – all change is challenging, particularly if you rely on routine and stability.

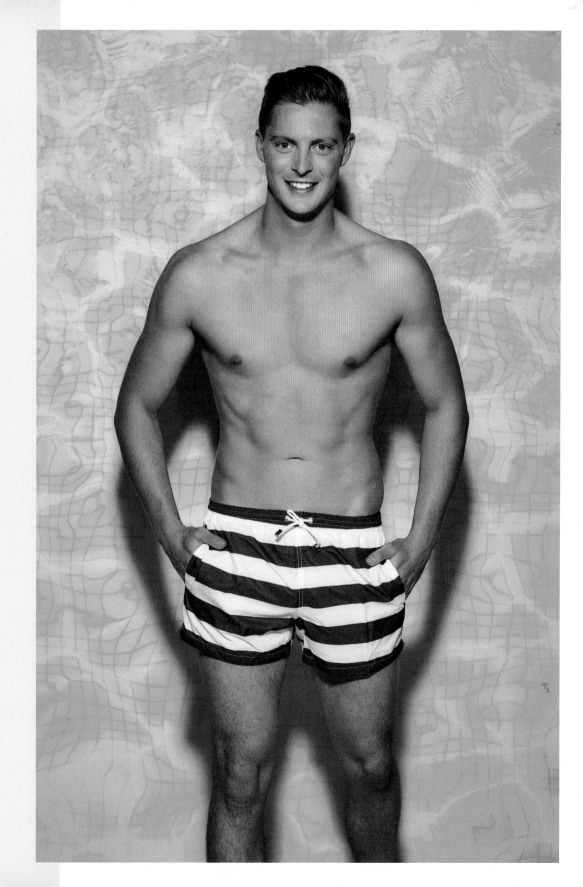

MENTAL HEALTH WAKE-UP CALL

I have always been someone who rolls with the punches; I tend to suppress my emotions and get on with things, which is strange when I consider how sensitive I actually am. However this stoicism became my undoing in my second year at medical school, when several things happened at once that shook me up and went on to have a lasting impact.

Firstly, as I talked about in Chapter 1, Freya, one of my closest friends, was diagnosed with leukaemia, which affected the friendship group we'd formed in the first year at med school. Secondly, just after we heard that news, the group was split up and scattered to different parts of Cornwall and Devon for our third year placement; I was sent to Truro and my girlfriend was placed in Exeter. Looking back, I think this was when I started to spiral. I was commuting back and forth to Exeter, trying to keep a long-distance relationship going, while being away from my friends in Truro, who were frustrated at my constant absence. To make matters worse, Freya was having her treatment in Plymouth, and I didn't feel I was pulling my weight supporting her there. And all the while I was trying to maintain my grades at medical school. I was spinning several plates at once and was in danger of having them all come crashing down around me.

It was a strange time, because I loved what I was doing – for the first three years my grades had been really good and medicine just clicked in a way nothing else ever had. But in my third year, my grades started to slip and so did my mental health. I felt very low, lost, lacking in motivation and extremely anxious all the time. I worried endlessly and excessively about my relationship, about Freya's illness, that I was losing my friendships and, in the end, it all became too much.

I started to isolate myself; I hardly saw my family and, in truth, I was actually very, very lonely. I stopped exercising, ate badly, didn't sleep, and stopped socializing or engaging in my usual hobbies. I was at a loss as to what to do and far too proud to ask for help. My reluctance to reach out was also compounded by my fear – unfounded, of course – that the medical school would look dimly on a soon-to-be doctor who was struggling with his mental health. I felt a real sense of shame and I was sure I would not be able to graduate if I was diagnosed with depression or anxiety.

WHEN TO SEEK HELP

It's always hard to pinpoint the best time to ask for help, because it differs from person to person. If we're honest with ourselves, I think we all know our trigger points, but it's often external factors that stop us from reaching out. Things to look out for in yourself or someone close to you include:

A lack of energy and motivation, even to do things previously found enjoyable

Feeling physically uncomfortable without any apparent cause

Change in appetite, either overeating or eating too little

Low or fluctuating mood

Difficulty getting to sleep and/or finding it hard to sleep well

Moving or speaking more slowly than usual

Low sex drive

The thought of asking for help made me feel sick, but I had to do something or I was simply going to break. So, finally, I asked my mum for help. I told her exactly how I felt, all of my worries and fears, my guilt and my angst and she listened. We spoke for hours on that first phone call and all of my suppressed emotion was released. Saying it out loud was a weight off my shoulders. It is hard to describe the relief I felt – it was immense. I slept better that night than I had in two years.

That phone call was a turning point for me. From there, I had the strength to tell my friends and my girlfriend how I felt, who, to my surprise, all told me they had realized there was something wrong. Together we came up with an action plan to make me feel better. We created an exercise programme and routine, and I planned healthy meals and timetabled work time and downtime. We allocated time in the week for socializing together and time to see my girlfriend. I even took up meditation, which was completely new to me. And Mum continued to speak to me on the phone every night for many months, which really helped.

Looking back, that first step of opening up was the tipping point; the cascade of change that followed started with that first crucial step. Over time I got better, and felt happier and healthier. The lessons I learned from that experience have proved invaluable for the things that have happened in the years since. Not least being in the spotlight on national TV.

My little brother and I often spoke about mental health, and I see my 'mental health toolkit' (opposite) as a legacy for Llŷr. But if you're struggling right now, there are also charities such as Samaritans, Mind and CALM ready to listen and help. Please reach out. There is always hope of a better day.

♥

SEVEN KEY ELEMENTS FOR GOOD MENTAL HEALTH

Even though I've had my fair share of 'dark times', I've tried to take those experiences and turn them into something positive. My 'mental health toolkit' – or protective interventions, if you prefer – is something I refer to constantly in order to maintain my mental and physical wellness.

There are several key aspects in which I believe we have to invest our time and energy in order to keep our mental wellbeing in check. They are routine, exercise, relationships, diet, sleep, mindfulness and perspective. I've touched upon all of these in the seven points below and this list should be referred to every time you're dealing with external stressors.

1. ROUTINE
Structure and routine in life form the blueprint for happiness. Make sure your days are varied and encompass the other key components to looking after both body and mind.

2. EXERCISE
Exercise for a healthy mind – do what you enjoy and what makes you feel good. You will be far more likely to stick at it and not give up (see Chapter 4).

3. TALK
As simple as it sounds, most of us don't do it enough. Talk to people you trust about the way you feel and be brave about sharing your feelings and emotions, in both the good and the bad times. This is vital for mental wellness.

4. MAKE TIME
Make time for things in life that make you happy, each and every day. Whether it is a walk, reading something by your favourite author or listening to music, invest in yourself and your happiness.

5. BELIEVE IN YOURSELF
Learn to love who you are – be your own biggest fan and remind yourself every day that what you are is enough. We are far too quick to bring ourselves down and compare ourselves harshly to others. Make sure to surround yourself with positive people, both in real life and on social media.

6. LIVE IN THE PRESENT
Nostalgia can be a wonderful thing, and looking back and remembering the good (and the not-so-good) times can be healthy and instructive. But a lot of people live their lives without being 'present'. Telling the voice in my brain to shut up and focus on the moment has helped me through some of my darkest times. There is only the now – this moment is the most important one, so live it.

7. MAKE SOCIAL MEDIA WORK FOR YOU
Social media has a lot going for it (you wouldn't be reading this book without it for a start), but if you allow it to get a hold of your life it can cause loss of perspective and feelings of isolation, which can lead to depression, anxiety and a loss of self-worth. To ensure this doesn't happen to you, look at the tips on page 57.

CHANGE AND MENTAL WELLNESS

When you look at your mental health as a whole, it's the big changes that happen in life that shine the light on how you feel overall. They don't necessarily have to be bad changes; even positive ones can unsettle you and cause reactions you didn't expect.

I remember when I was at school and I thought that life would be straightforward, a series of steps that would lead naturally from one to the next. What I've come to realize is that life takes you in many directions. Sometimes we can influence the journey, sometimes we can't. Life is not linear and change will happen, for good or bad.

Accepting that things change is an important part of dealing with it – resisting change can actually hinder the process. It's better to accept that change is happening and then look at

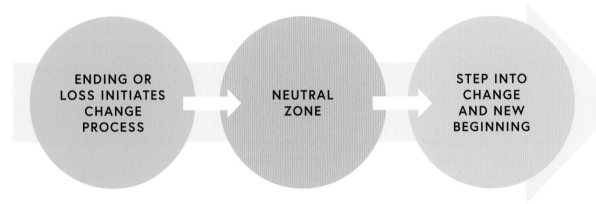

ENDING OR LOSS INITIATES CHANGE PROCESS

NEUTRAL ZONE

STEP INTO CHANGE AND NEW BEGINNING

At the beginning of the change process as described in the Bridges Transition Model, there might be strong emotions or heightened reactions

Before change occurs, there is period of uncertainty when you might feel resentment or apathy towards change – this is completely natural

Once change is processed and accepted, you can embrace it with renewed energy and openness to the potential

which other aspects of your life you can keep the same. Can you still exercise? Can you still eat healthily? Can you still find time for yourself and your loved ones? If you can stick to at least part of your pre-change routine, it means that there are some parts of your life that are staying the same. Of course if it's an all-encompassing change like a bereavement, then that is something else entirely, but still simple things such as being active can go a long way.

And as always, don't be afraid to ask for help, whether it's from a friend, family member or an organization. There are people out there who will listen and not judge you. Change is like a pebble thrown into a still pond: no matter what size the stone, there are bound to be ripples. Knowing this will help us ride out those ripples as best we can and get back to the placid water again.

ANTI-DEPRESSANTS

Treating depression always requires a multi-faceted approach. It could involve lifestyle changes, such as diet and exercise, talking therapies, such as counselling and lifestyle coaching, or taking medication like anti-depressants. One of the most common things I hear people worrying about when it comes to anti-depressants is that anti-depressants will turn them into a different person or that any happiness they feel will be false, just a product of the medication. Anti-depressants work by restoring the balance of mood hormones in your brain, which for some may be out of sync. They also give you the mental energy you need to make changes to your life, which ultimately will make you happier. Some are afraid they will become reliant on them, unable to stop taking them once started. In actual fact, most people will be able to come off their medication after the prescribed period of time, aided by careful guidance and planning from their doctor. Don't get me wrong, a pill is not a quick fix. But alongside other changes to your life, and combined with talking therapies, they can really help you in your journey to finding equilibrium again.

MY EXPERIENCE: SOCIAL MEDIA

Most things in life are a mixture of good and bad and social media is no different. It has loads of positives – it can be inspirational, supportive, empowering and can create communities. However, it is open to misuse too, and sometimes the downsides can seem to outweigh the benefits, causing untold amounts of stress, upset and anxiety.

I appreciate that my experience is far from typical, but I think it's allowed me to see social media at its very best, as well as its very worst. As with most *Love Island* contestants, appearing on the show gave my social media following a massive boost. As I said in Chapter 1, this was an incredible platform from which to give an insight into life in a busy NHS A&E department and, since the start of the Covid-19 pandemic, I have helped to spread important public health messages via my channels on YouTube and Instagram. It seemed to me the ideal use of my ability to reach such a big audience.

Of course, there will always be trolls, but on the whole I think I've dealt with them fairly well. I have a relatively thick skin, which is handy considering how much I was trolled for my sunburn on *Love Island*! That was my first experience of deliberately offensive and unkind comments on such a large scale and I was shocked at how brutal people could be; people who didn't know me or my personal situation accused me of being a bad doctor, irresponsible, uneducated and reckless, all because I got sunburned! In truth, I was taking isotretinoin, a medication to treat acne, which happens to make your skin incredibly sensitive and therefore turn pink in the sun more easily. Nothing to do with lack of factor 50! This experience taught me two great lessons. Don't let the narration of others define who you are. And never, ever, feed the trolls.

It's my belief that those who take shots at me on social media are almost always doing so from a position of jealousy or weakness. I heard a great saying once – 'Whoever is trying to bring you down is already below you.' Jealousy is a truly terrible trait; there is no winner where jealousy is involved. I have learned to separate and distance myself both mentally and physically from people with this characteristic. Believe me, your stress levels will diminish the minute you cut people like this out of your life – real or virtual!

Managing your social media

Start by monitoring how long and in what way you spend time online. Be honest, are you whiling away hours on social media? If so, try to limit how long you spend online

Keep your phone in another room when you're watching TV or spending time with friends and family

Curate your feeds properly – follow positive accounts only and unfollow negative ones or those that engender negative feelings (including jealousy)

Ensure you have downtime and plan for phone-free periods (Sunday mornings are a good one)

Remember that social media itself is curated; it's not reality, it's 'life' carefully filtered and presented in a particular way, with all the awkward edges smoothed off. And everything that you see is already in the past – click 'like' and move on

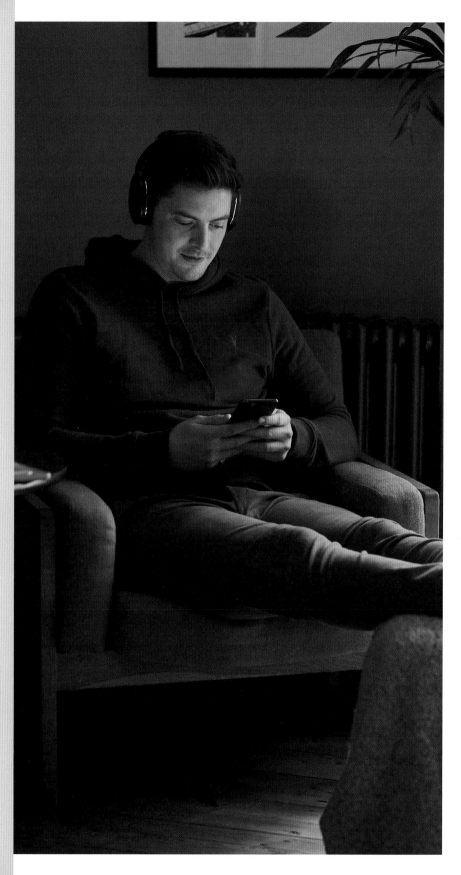

The only time when trolling does get to me, because I am human and a sensitive one at that, is when colleagues in the medical profession have a dig. I am, however, fortunate and incredibly grateful that I also receive a lot of support from colleagues across the NHS, as well as in the hospital where I work.

As hard as you might try, you can never please everybody. When I lost my brother last year, I decided to take some time out from social media. For a couple of months I focused on my family, my work and my own mental health. During that time there were a few unbelievably hurtful comments aimed at me, but for the most part the support I got was incredibly supportive and moving. I'm not exaggerating when I tell you I received hundreds of thousands of messages of kindness and care, for both me and my family, and every single one made a real difference. When I started posting on my channels again, the response was overwhelming.

So while social media gets a bad rep, I tend to focus on the positives and the amazing things it can do. Used correctly it be an incredible tool for good. So let's be the change we want to see and continue using it in that way.

The strength of our connections with family, friends and colleagues has a huge impact on our mental health – something I think we all learned from the Covid-19 pandemic. Social media enables us to reach out, to maintain and nurture our relationships, and this can ease stress, provide joy and boost self-esteem.

DEALING WITH STRESS

'I'm stressed out!' It's a phrase we're all familiar with and one I'm sure we've all said at some point. But what do we really mean when we say it? A medical dictionary would say that stress is the body's reaction to any change that requires an adjustment or response. And those responses can be physical, mental and emotional.

Different people have different ways of reacting to stress. One person's threshold can be higher than another's; some people thrive under pressure, others find it difficult. Regardless of where you are on the scale, a 2018 report from the Mental Health Foundation found that 74 per cent of people in the UK have experienced levels of stress that made them feel overwhelmed or unable to cope. That's a pretty large percentage – it seems we're a stressed nation and that's not good for our mental health. But we cannot avoid stress – life happens – and it's how we deal with those challenges that defines us.

As I've talked about earlier, my life challenges have been varied. It goes without saying that the job of a doctor can be very stressful – we are confronting life and death every day. A&E is busy and there is a lot to juggle. But to do my job well I need to be able to handle my stress levels, as well as find time to decompress once I've finished my shift, whether it's been a particularly stressful one or not. And I'm sure the same is true for you – you don't have to be a doctor working in A&E to be stressed out by the challenges thrown at you. It's not letting those challenges overcome us that matters. It's all about having a strong foundation for mental resilience and using such challenges – stressors – to create success and personal development rather than failure.

Our mood impacts everything we do or even *try* to do. If you think about it, phrases like 'duvet day' all stem from the idea that there are times when we simply can't face the world and want to hide away. A strong mindset is vital for a balanced and healthy lifestyle, but there are many things that can stop the mind from functioning at full capacity. The key is to recognize the ways in which we can help ourselves and look after our mental function, in exactly the same way we would any other organ or body part. Stress and poor mental health are definitely something to take as seriously as any other illness we need to manage.

**MAKING SMALL CHANGES TO THE WAY YOU
APPROACH THINGS WILL ENSURE YOU'RE BETTER
PREPARED FOR WHAT LIFE THROWS AT YOU.**

IDENTIFYING CHALLENGES

For me, this is about identifying if what I'm feeling is temporary or whether it's a sign of a larger issue. I know what I need to do to ensure I stay on top of things – eat healthily, exercise, have time to decompress – and a good indication that things are getting on top of me is if I stop doing those things, which of course exacerbates the problem. This is my 'early warning system' and I've included this as part of my top stress-busting tips on the following pages.

As long as you have breath in your lungs, challenges will continue to come. The key is to be self-aware and manage the stressors before they overwhelm you and tip you into experiencing depressive or hopeless feelings. I experience a lot of potentially stressful situations at work daily and, if I let every single case get to me, would I be a good and objective doctor? Absolutely not. I would be a wreck in the corner and would almost certainly quit. Being able to realize that you have done everything you can and accepting your limitations are so important in dealing with what life throws at you. Do your best and know that that is enough.

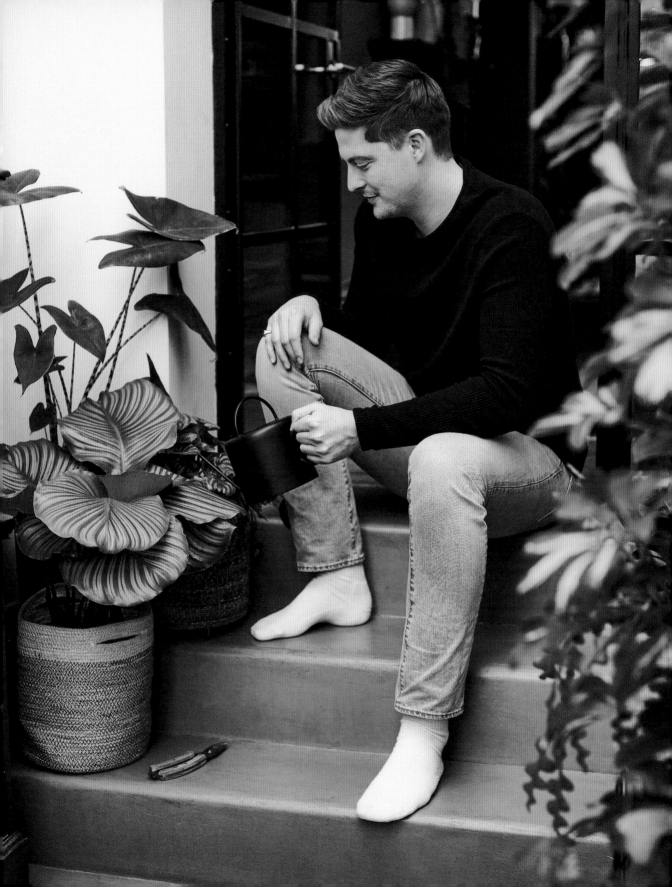

SEVEN TIPS FOR DEALING WITH STRESS

1. Get some perspective

Give your stress a value. If you see this as a big problem, compare it to other ones. Do you know of other people who have overcome greater adversity? Ask yourself, 'Am I making a mountain out of a molehill?' Asking and answering these questions out loud will often bring you to the conclusion that things aren't that bad and that, even if they are, you will still get through it.

2. Deal with stress straight away

If you put off dealing with a challenge it will become a problem. Break it down. What is causing the stress? Is it actually a problem? For example, maybe you have moved to a new town, with all the worry that comes with finding somewhere to live, and are wondering whether you will make friends. Often, if you reframe a problem, you find out it's actually a massive opportunity. Say to yourself, 'I get to move to experience a different environment, find a beautiful new home and meet wonderful people.'

3. Create targets and write a list

Write down everything you can do to overcome the situation. I emphasize 'everything you can do', because you should only consider things inside your sphere of influence. If you can't control it, don't waste mental energy on it. Once you have your list, try to tick off everything on it. Know that you've done all you can do.

4. Talk it through

When it comes to stress, talking is the best medicine you can prescribe yourself. Whether it was my mum when I was at med school or the producers after I left *Love Island*, when I was feeling overwhelmed, I turned to others for help. If you're having work issues, speak to a line manager or your HR department; if your stress is more personal, then a friend or sibling may surprise you by how good a listener they can be. It's worth reiterating that Samaritans, Mind and CALM have trained staff ready to listen. And don't forget your GP, who can give you options you may not know are available.

5. Be good to yourself

When I've experienced low moods in the past, the first things to go are the things that would probably help me the most. Core life elements such as exercise, eating healthily and getting enough sleep, all proven to help with anxiety and depression, fall by the wayside as stress takes hold. Exercise in particular is a big part of managing my stress. Sometimes it's so hard to exercise when I feel tired and stressed, but it is the best thing I can do to feel better. Even doing short workouts for 15–20 minutes in the kitchen is important for body and mind, particularly if stress is making it hard for you to leave the house. Paying attention to your nutrition is vital too – feeding your mind and body properly can really help you manage dark spells and negative cycles.

6. Learn to say no

We can all find reasons not to say no to something. You may think you'll be letting people down or you'll upset someone. At work you may feel you have a duty to your colleagues to take on that extra workload or you may worry people will think you're a shirker or lazy if you don't. But the main reason people find it hard to say no is that they simply don't know how to. One look at my diary and you'll see I'm one of them! But it is important to learn how to say no and the best way to do that is literally to practise saying the word out loud. And don't feel that you have to be nice when saying no – polite yes, but don't feel you have to apologize. There's nothing to be sorry about when you're taking positive steps to reduce your stress levels and improve your mental health.

7. Find time for something you love

Remember when we talked about a 360-degree approach to health? Well, doing something you love is part of that big picture. When you're overburdened with stress, particularly of the work kind, taking time to do something you enjoy can seem frivolous and unimportant. But studies have found that engaging in leisure activities can actively reduce the stress from other areas of our lives, as well as boost overall mood. I love driving fast cars and getting out for a track day is my ideal way of unwinding (I know – hardly relaxing you might think!). But I also love going for a bike ride to clear my head and get some exercise. Whether it's sport, gardening, painting or cooking, taking time out for yourself away from the source of your stress is one of the best things you can do.

MEN AND MENTAL HEALTH

The biggest misconceptions

Mental health only affects the 'weak-minded' and it makes you less 'manly'

It can't happen to me

Those who are successful and wealthy are immune

If you have poor mental health, it will never be good again

Lifestyle changes don't work

Top three things men worry about most in relation to being honest about their mental health

Stigma, by far – men are afraid of being judged for their mental health

That it will affect their careers and ability to progress in life

Opening up – men are much less likely to talk about their feelings or ask for help

Mental health affects everyone. Anyone can experience poor mental health and therefore everyone should be looking after their own wellbeing and that of those around them.

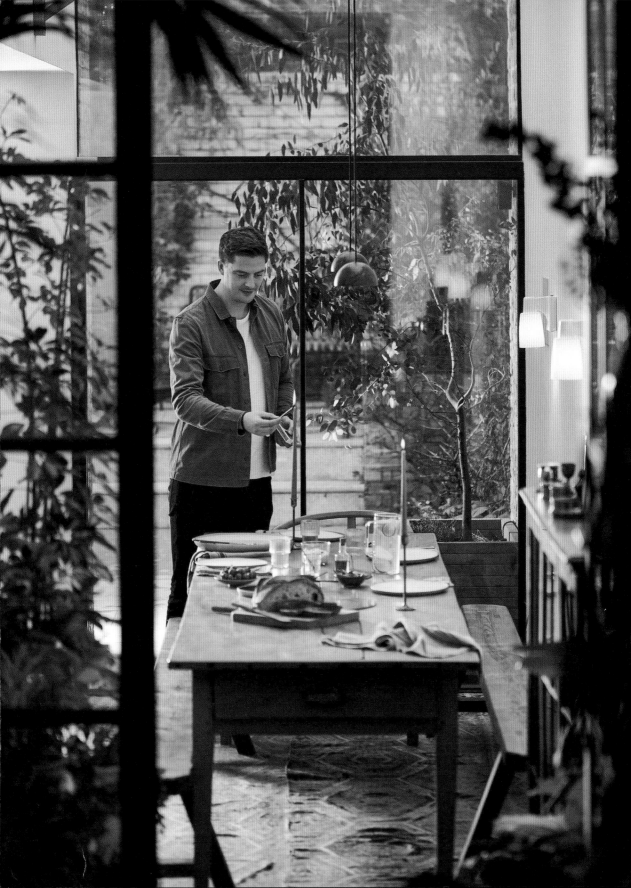

TAKE A MENTAL HEALTH INVENTORY

I believe one of the most important things when it comes to positive mental health is knowing yourself. Being aware of where you are in life, what's working for you and what isn't, is essential for avoiding stressful situations that may cause undue anxiety or worse.

Taking a mental health inventory is like any form of diarizing or journalling; the process of doing it is useful in itself. Making the time to look inward, having a good think about how you're really feeling and then externalizing those feelings by writing them down can be a powerful tool for avoiding stressors, or at least knowing how to handle them when you do encounter them.

It doesn't have to be an ongoing thing, but it can be useful if you find yourself in a situation you've struggled with historically. All you need to do is sit down with a pen and a pad of paper and start by answering the following seven questions:

1. **Are you getting enough quality sleep? If not, what's keeping you awake?**

2. **Are you managing stress well? What mechanisms are you using to cope?**

3. **Are you getting out of the house every day? Are you exercising?**

4. **Are you eating healthily? When was the last time you made a meal from scratch?**

5. **Are you doing things you enjoy? When was the last time you did an activity that made you happy?**

6. **Are you getting satisfaction from your work? Do you feel useful?**

7. **When was the last time you told someone how you feel? Could you pick up the phone and do that right now?**

Look at your answers. In some areas you may feel like you're doing OK, but in others you may not. For example, during a busy week in A&E I might be feeling good about myself, getting out of the house and sleeping well (because I'm exhausted!), but could be falling down on the healthy eating and doing things I enjoy. So I try to focus on those. You can use the other chapters in this book to give you pointers on how to improve in the areas you're not happy with. The physical influences the mental, and vice versa, so cooking yourself a healthy meal and then going out for an evening walk can do wonders for your mood and self-esteem, as well as your overall health.

The main thing though, is taking the time out to have a think about yourself and how you're actually feeling. It may sound simple, but reconnecting with ourselves is one of the most important things we can do when it comes to our mental health and happiness.

WHAT CAN YOU DO TODAY?

GET OUTSIDE

Take immediate positive action and go for a walk. Get some fresh air, feel the sun on your face (or the rain, it doesn't matter) and move your body. Honestly, I walk all the time and it's my number one health tip – mental or physical. Walk, move, breathe. And be present. Don't think about what you've done or what you've got to do – just be in the moment, because that moment is 100 per cent yours.

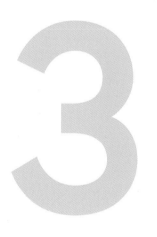

3 THE KEY TO A HEALTHY RELATIONSHIP WITH FOOD IS EATING TO FEEL GOOD, NOT LOOK GOOD. CHOOSE MORE PLANT-BASED FOODS, GIVE YOUR GUT HEALTH A BOOST AND EAT MINDFULLY.

NUTRITION

I was going to call this chapter Eat Well Every Day, but none of us is perfect, least of all me. I've learned, however, that if we know the basics of nutrition, it makes healthy choices come naturally. If we eat to fuel ourselves and feel good, rather than to comfort ourselves or look good, that's a healthier relationship with food right there.

My aim in this chapter is to reassure you that you don't have to spend your life on a diet. Yes, good nutrition matters – it has a huge impact on how you feel day to day, as well as your long-term health – but it's not something you need to obsess about. You don't need to tick all of the boxes, all of the time.

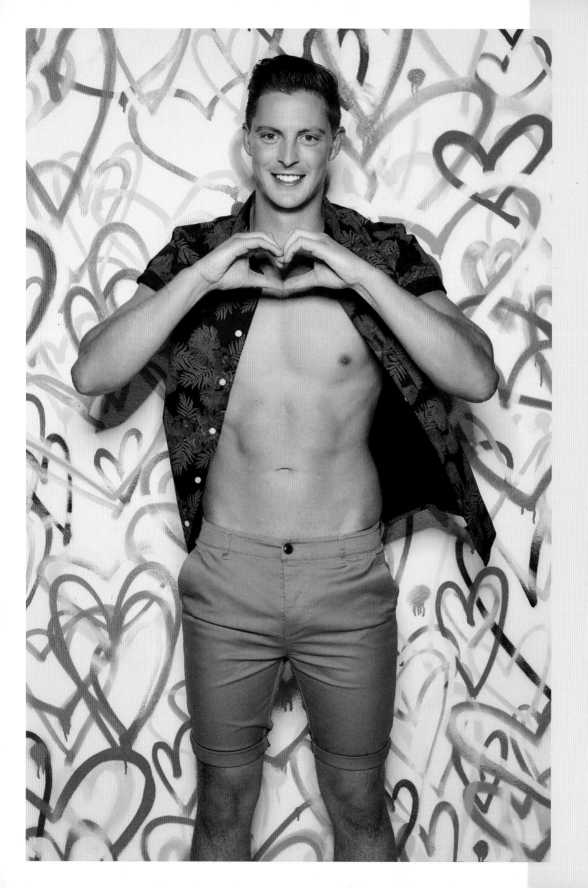

MY EXPERIENCE:
LOVE ISLAND LOOKS

The food and drink we consume on a regular basis have the power both to heal and to damage us. They can nourish or punish. And the same goes for what we choose *not* to eat or drink. Sounds simple, but it took me a while to work this out.

When looking at my own relationship with food, an obvious stage of my life to analyse is just before I went on *Love Island*. It was such a complicated time and the thought of being on TV will plunge even the most confident person into a vortex of self-doubt. All I could think about was being on screen without many clothes and how I would look. I was fit and cycled to work every day, but it didn't feel like enough. So I embarked on a 20-week diet and training regime to 'transform' my physique. I wanted to look as good as possible.

My diet was strict: I started denying myself certain foods and avoided any situation that might tempt me to fall off the wagon. This meant that I stopped going out, stopped seeing my friends. I watched my body get leaner, but I became less and less healthy. By the time the show start date was approaching, I was barely eating. What I *was* eating was just food to bulk up on muscle and cut down my fat percentage. I was motivated by aesthetics not health. My meals were functional, often processed, rarely tasty. I'm talking protein shakes, bars, you know the sort of thing. Having learned more now, I wouldn't call my diet then nutritious. I felt terrible; I was tired, moody and obsessive when it came to my training.

My constant obsession with my body created and compounded an unhealthy mindset and habit so that, by the time I was on the show, lean physique notwithstanding, I just felt incredibly self-conscious. The fact my skin was red upset me no end, and I felt I wasn't in good enough shape or good-looking enough to be there.

Now, I know I was in a very small minority of people who find (or put!) themselves in the public eye. But I'm sharing this because I think lots of you have felt or feel the same. That pressure to look a certain way, whether it's for work, your social media feed, in front of your friends or potential partners, it doesn't matter. My message to you is: please, don't punish yourself like I did. If what you're eating doesn't make you feel alive and energized, if constantly tracking what you eat is taking over your life, then I hope this chapter can be the reality check – and the source of real, valuable nutrition information – you need.

**REMEMBER: NOURISH, DON'T PUNISH.
ENRICH, DON'T RESTRICT.**

EAT TO FEEL GOOD, NOT LOOK GOOD

I'm really pleased to report that I think this message is already getting through. Lots of the messages I receive from people on Instagram suggest that people want to understand more about eating well and exercising right. They're savvy about the false promise of fad diets and quick-fix weight-loss or bulking products. As a doctor this is music to my ears!

It might seem like a small change, but pre-*Love Island* me certainly didn't come across much evidence of this sensible thinking. The loudest conversations on social media just a few years ago were all about the fastest ways to change your body composition and make sure your abs showed.

I think a good relationship with food means looking at is as something that creates energy and health, seeing it as friend not foe. Food is fuel. My experience leading up to *Love Island* taught me that, whether for athletic performance or simply going about our daily lives, we should look at food as a source of vitality.

OK, that's not a green light to eat absolutely everything and anything. Malnutrition is defined as, 'lack of proper nutrition, caused by not having enough to eat, not eating enough of the right things, or being unable to use the food that one does eat.' In other words, you can be overweight and malnourished. A healthy, balanced diet, essentially, is eating the right quantity of the right things to fuel and maintain our bodies properly.

These days, I understand that what I put on my plate, along with how and when I eat it, has a massive impact on how I feel and how I cope with stress. A busy lifestyle isn't an excuse to forget about good nutrition – in fact, it's a reason to learn more about it. You only get one body, so celebrate and nurture it because it has a big job to do. How? It's honestly simpler than you might think…

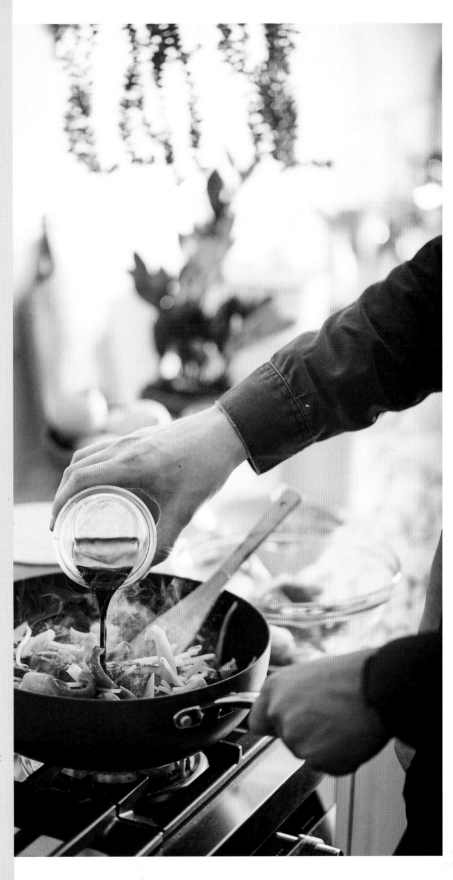

11

signs you might have an unhealthy relationship with food

Constant fluctuations in weight

Being overly fixated with your weight or body shape

Avoiding social situations due to food restrictions

Not wanting to eat in front of people

Eating when not hungry or not eating when you are

Never allowing yourself a 'treat' or 'unhealthy' meal

Eliminating entire categories of food

Not being truthful about what you have or haven't eaten

No longer getting enjoyment from food

Making yourself sick or hiding food

Linking your self-esteem to how well you stick to a diet

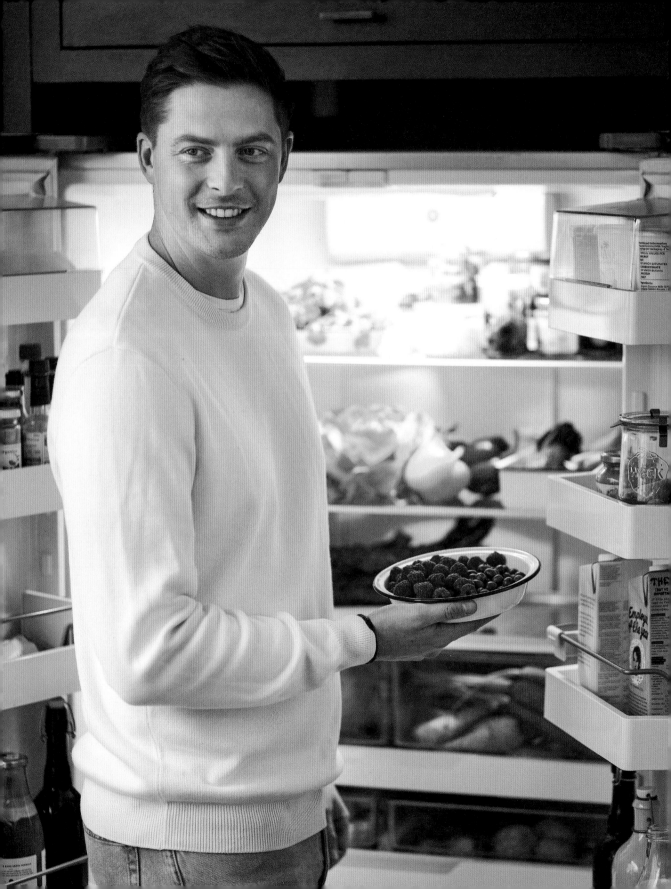

BACK TO NUTRITION BASICS

I don't expect you to become an expert in the subject, but a decent understanding of nutrition is essential for everyday health. It's something I've had to learn for myself because, believe it or not, you get precious little training on healthy eating in medical school.

You'd think it would be a really important subject for medical professionals, wouldn't you? After all, diet directly impacts both long- and short-term health. But unless your healthcare professional chooses to specialize in nutrition, chances are they don't know a huge amount more than you do. So here's my quick guide to what I think it's useful to know.

You might have heard the term 'macronutrients' when it comes to talking about diet (people in the fitness world often talk about counting 'macros'). They're essentially the three main groups we divide foods into: carbohydrates, fats and protein. And they're all vital for our bodies to function properly. Be wary of any diet that cuts out or significantly restricts one of these three macros – it may not be good for you. You need a balance.

During digestion, our bodies break carbohydrates down into sugars, fats into fatty acids and protein into amino acids, and then we're able to absorb and make use of them. Most foods contain more than one macro. Vegetables are carbohydrates, but still contain protein. Meat is a protein, but still contains fat. We don't eat single nutrients, we eat real food (or we should – manufacturers of meal-replacement shakes take note).

If you think you might be developing a disordered eating pattern, it's important to talk to someone and get advice before it escalates. You don't have to be a certain weight or look a certain way to have an eating disorder. Please talk to your GP or try some of the organizations listed on page 233).

WHAT DO THE MACRONUTRIENTS DO FOR ME?

- Carbohydrates provide energy. This group includes complex or non-digestible carbs, aka dietary fibre, which feed gut microbes, regulate your bowels and reduce the risk of heart disease and Type 2 diabetes. Simple carbs are found in: bread, rice, potatoes, pasta, cereals, plus the naturally occurring sugars in veg, fruit and milk. Complex carbs are in: wholegrains, legumes, vegetables and fruit, nuts and seeds.
- Fats provide essential fatty acids, as well as energy. We need fats to maintain the normal structure of cells in our body, as well as for skin health and immunity. Fats also help absorption of fat-soluble vitamins. They are found in: fats and oils, meat, oily fish, dairy, nuts and seeds, and avocados.
- Protein is essential for your muscles and skeleton, and also provides energy. Protein is found in: meat, fish, eggs, dairy, cereal products, soya products (like tofu), legumes, nuts and seeds.

MEGA MICRONUTRIENTS

'Micronutrients' are all the vitamins and minerals that are essential for good health. There's plenty of information available on what different vitamins and minerals can do for your health (reliable sources include the British Dietetic Association's Food Fact Sheets, the British Nutrition Foundation and the NHS). Lots of them work in synergy with each other – vitamin C helps your body absorb iron, for example. So don't think taking vitamin and mineral supplements can make up for a poor diet. They have their place if someone has a deficiency, but food always comes first.

All sorts of other helpful chemicals and compounds are released when our bodies start to break down food. Think different types of fibre that feed our gut microbes (more on them later) and omega-3 essential fatty acids that have an anti-inflammatory action. Plant foods are packed with antioxidants and plant chemicals like polyphenols that have health-promoting properties. A lot of plant chemicals are found in the pigments of plants, which give them their colour. So by 'eating the rainbow' you up the range of valuable plant chemicals you're consuming. And once again, they all act in synergy with each other.

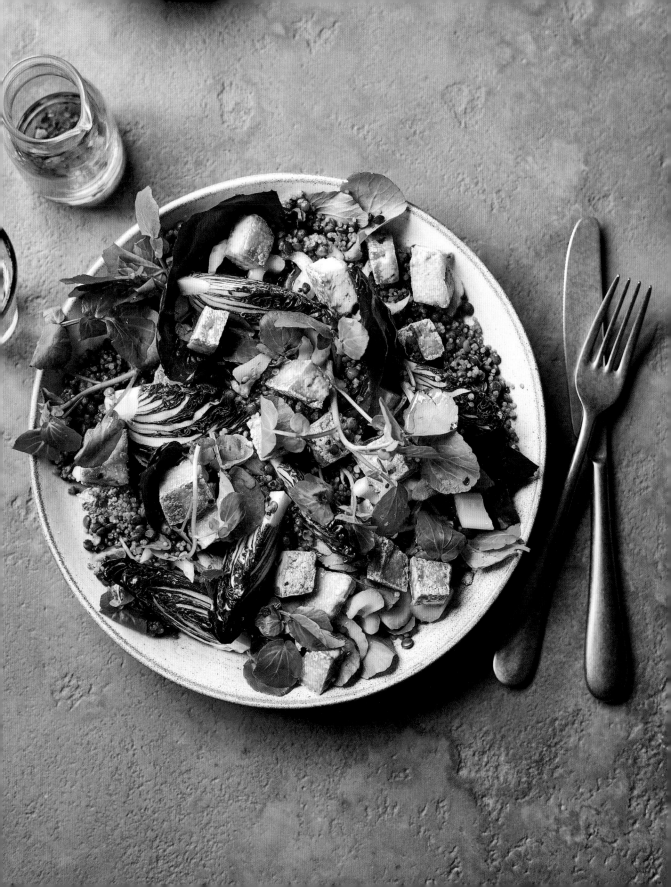

OUR BODIES ARE DESIGNED TO GET ALL NUTRIENTS FROM FOOD, NOT VITAMIN AND MINERAL SUPPLEMENTS.

THE EATWELL GUIDE

So you need all these nutrients, but how many? The government and NHS Eatwell Guide is a good starting point for advice. It divides up the food groups on a plate, so you can visualize what should be on yours.

Fill one-third of your plate with vegetables, salad or fruit. Fresh, tinned, frozen, dried, it doesn't matter – you've probably heard of eating your 'five-a-day' and that should be your minimum.

Another third of your plate should be starchy carbohydrates. That's your bread, pasta, rice, potatoes, cereals and other grains. Go for wholegrain varieties wherever possible.

The next biggest section on your plate is for protein. The advice is to eat less red and processed meat, more legumes (lentils, beans, chickpeas, etc) and, if you eat fish, to have two portions a week, one of which is oily. This section also includes poultry and eggs.

Finally, add some dairy, such as milk, yogurt and cheese, or fortified dairy alternatives (fortified meaning they have the nutrients you'd find in dairy added to them, like calcium). Choose lower fat where available. Then include small amounts of unsaturated oils, fats and spreads, like olive and rapeseed oil.

And while they don't make it to the plate itself, there is a little room in your diet for those foods (and drinks) that are high in salt, sugar or fat – cakes, crisps, juices, fizzy drinks, condiments and so on. These don't add anything useful to our diets but we're not all perfect all the time. As long as these make up a small proportion of your intake and the rest is healthy on a regular basis, it's fine to include them as occasional treats.

Personally, I wouldn't panic about making every meal you eat look like this plate. It's just a guide to what a balanced diet looks like – so aim for these sort of proportions over a week.

FRUIT & VEGETABLES

eat at least five portions
of a variety of fruit and
vegetables every day

POTATOES, BREAD, RICE, PASTA & OTHER STARCHY CARBOHYDRATES

choose wholegrain or higher
fibre versions with less added
fats, salt and sugar

BEANS, PULSES, FISH, EGGS, MEAT & OTHER PROTEINS

eat more beans and pulses,
two portions of sustainably sourced
fish per week, one of which is oily.
Eat less red and processed meat

DAIRY & ALTERNATIVES

choose lower-fat and
lower-sugar options

OILS & SPREADS

choose unsaturated
oils and use in
small amounts

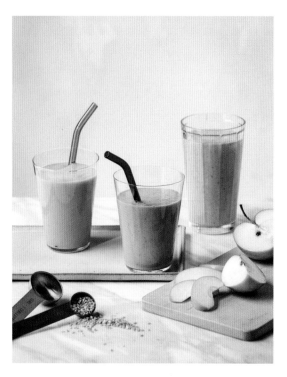

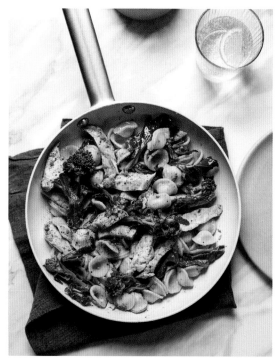

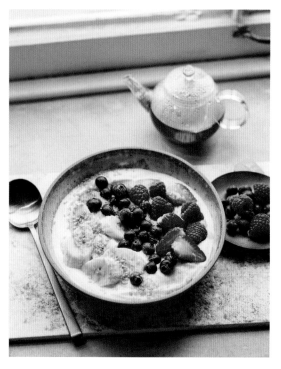

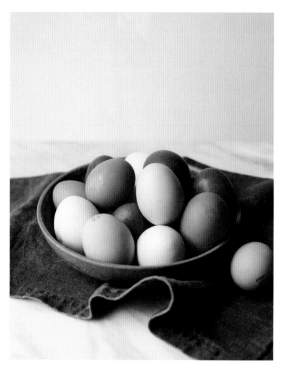

WEIGHTY ISSUES

When it comes to weight loss or maintaining a healthy weight (more on this in Chapter 4), I'm not going to endorse any diet 'tribe' or fad. I'm a big believer that if you stick to the sort of healthy eating guidelines described already, and you take regular exercise, your 'happy' weight won't be too far out of reach. Of course, there are other factors that contribute – stress, medication, even those gut microbes I keep mentioning. My point is stay away from quick-fix diets, products and supplements.

Of course, it's important not to carry too much weight. Obesity is linked with Type 2 diabetes, coronary artery disease, some cancers, stroke and musculoskeletal disorders – and it certainly lowers resilience to other diseases and conditions, as the Covid-19 pandemic has shown. Globally, rates have tripled since 1975. This is endangering the health of a huge number of people. And yet it's potentially preventable.

I could spend pages here going into all the latest research on various different diets – low-carb, high-protein, low-fat, no-fat, *high*-fat, fasting, grazing, juicing – only to conclude that a) different things work for different people and b) nothing extreme is often healthy or sustainable in the long run. What I think does help is to have a basic idea of energy in versus energy out. Going back to my analogy of food as fuel, any food your body doesn't use up as fuel will be stored as fat. So we need to aim for a balance of eating and activity.

You will all have heard of calories, which are the energy measurement for food. The average man needs 2,500 calories a day and the average woman requires 2,000. But, if you want to lose weight, it's suggested you cut this by around 500 calories a day and increase your activity levels to match. Of course, to know how many calories you're consuming, you'll need to know how many are in each food. You can work this out from food labels (see page 83) or use the NHS calorie checker or an app like MyFitnessPal or Nutracheck (see Resources, page 233, for more information). Some are really sophisticated and let you scan barcodes with your phone, others are a database of common, generic foods.

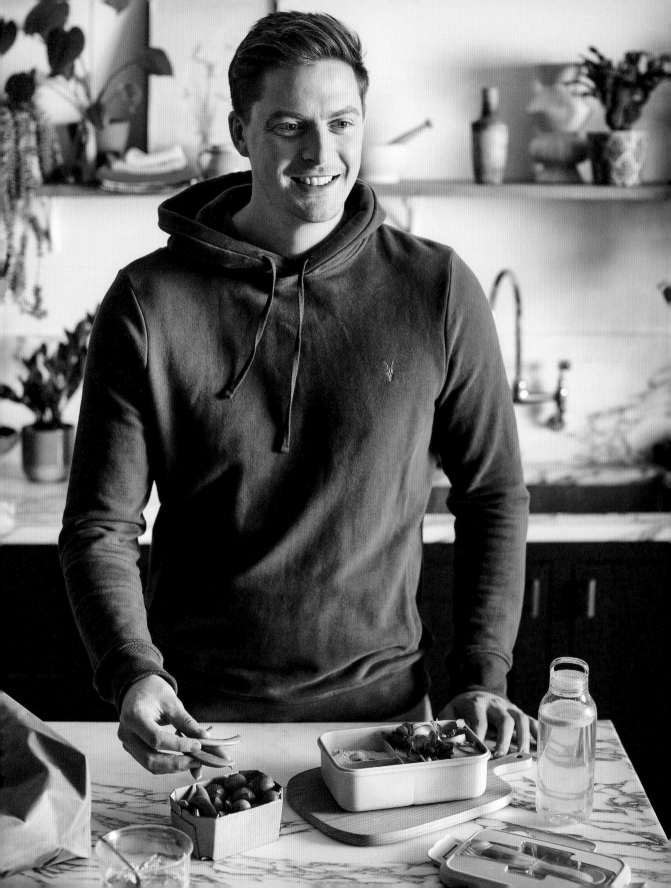

Calorie counting is pretty controversial these days. While it's still the NHS and government's solution for weight loss, there are lots of experts who say it's inaccurate and irrelevant – that it doesn't take into account the nutrient value of the food, which is true. I would add the criticism that it can become obsessive. If you spend every mealtime reading labels, fiddling on your phone and weighing portions, it takes all the pleasure out of eating.

My advice? I think it's really handy to check in with yourself and get an honest picture of what you typically eat in a day. Tracking your food and calorie intake over a few days can also be an education, in a 'Wow, *how* many calories are in that cereal bar?' sort of way that can prompt you to make some healthier choices easily. Often you'll find simple wins – skip that mid-morning croissant and afternoon biscuit break and that's 500 calories cut right there. Just make sure you don't become a slave to your apps. It's not all about the numbers.

HOW TO READ A FOOD LABEL

All packaged foods have an ingredients label on the side. It's worth checking these to keep tabs on what's really healthy. Here are my tips:

- Ingredients are listed in order of weight, so whatever comes first on the list is what the product contains most of. If sugar, fat or salt are high up on that list, it's not a healthy food.
- Likewise, if a product says it has a certain healthy ingredient in it, check how far up the list that ingredient is. It might only have a tiny amount!
- If an ingredients list is very long, with lots of chemical names you don't understand, it's an ultra-processed food and best avoided.
- Sugar hides on labels in lots of forms. Look for fructose, maltose, dextrose – basically anything ending in -ose – as well as syrups and honey.
- Check the packaging for the traffic-light labelling system. Foods are given green, amber or red logos depending on how high they are in sugar, saturated fat and salt. Green's the best choice, save red for treats.
- If you're comparing calories or fat for different foods, make sure you're looking at the same amounts. Food labels break down each nutrient by overall weight of the product, sometimes by suggested portion size and by 100g. I tend to look at the 100g column.

SWITCH THINGS UP: VARIETY IS IMPORTANT IN A HEALTHY, BALANCED DIET.

WHAT DO I EAT?

Individual nutritional needs vary from person to person. Here's an example, however, of what I normally eat during the day to stay energized, motivated and feeling healthy. I try to keep it simple: three meals a day with the odd healthy snack, but only if I need it to keep me going. This is for a day when I'm not on shift in A&E (when, try as I might, meals often don't go to plan). Of course, I enjoy the occasional treat, but I try to stick to this pattern of eating as much as possible.

My mindset is that an unhealthy meal or snack isn't a problem, it's the unhealthy *diet* that's the issue – the food that makes up the majority of your intake on a regular basis. Another way of looking at it is the 80:20 split. Aim for 80 per cent of your diet to be healthy and balanced, so 20 per cent can be more relaxed.

Depending on my shift patterns, I switch up some of the above. If I'm getting up to do a bicycle ride before work, I have some quick carbs (like a banana) and, when I get back for breakfast, I make sure I have some slow-release carbs like porridge. As the name suggests, they release their energy gradually (unlike, say, a sugary drink) to fuel the day. I'm a big fan of nuts too – they are a great source of healthy fats and proteins to help my body recover from exercise.

When I'm on shift during the day, I make sure I have some lighter foods, such as a small bowl of brown pasta, tuna and salad, to keep my energy levels up. Water is key throughout the day. At night, after work, having plenty of protein helps me feel full, and also starts to get my body to unwind and feel ready for sleep.

BREAKFAST	Yogurt with banana and blueberries with a cup of coffee	This is a good mixture of vitamins, fats and carbohydrates for energy. Caffeine has a stimulant effect and aids concentration.
LUNCH	Pasta with chicken and broccoli	I aim for a good balance of carbs, fats and protein. Often by midday our energy levels drop and the slow-release carb gives a welcome boost for the rest of the day.
DINNER	Tuna and mixed salad with a yogurt dessert	In the evening, energy-giving carbohydrates are often less important (unless a night shift is looming); instead proteins, which aid in satiety and recovery, as well as healthy fats, take priority.

7 SNACKS I ALWAYS
HAVE AT WORK

The key here is to keep healthy snacks with you – in your desk,
locker, bag, glove box – so you don't get caught out and head
for the vending machine.

Bananas, oranges, apples or other fruit

Nuts, such as almonds – rich in good fats, complex carbohydrates and protein

Granola bars for slow-release energy (check the label as some are high in sugar)

A can of tuna in spring water or a hard-boiled egg – some protein to fill me up

Natural yogurt for protein and fat (and gut health – more on this later!)

Veggie crudités and hummus

Peanut butter on oatcakes

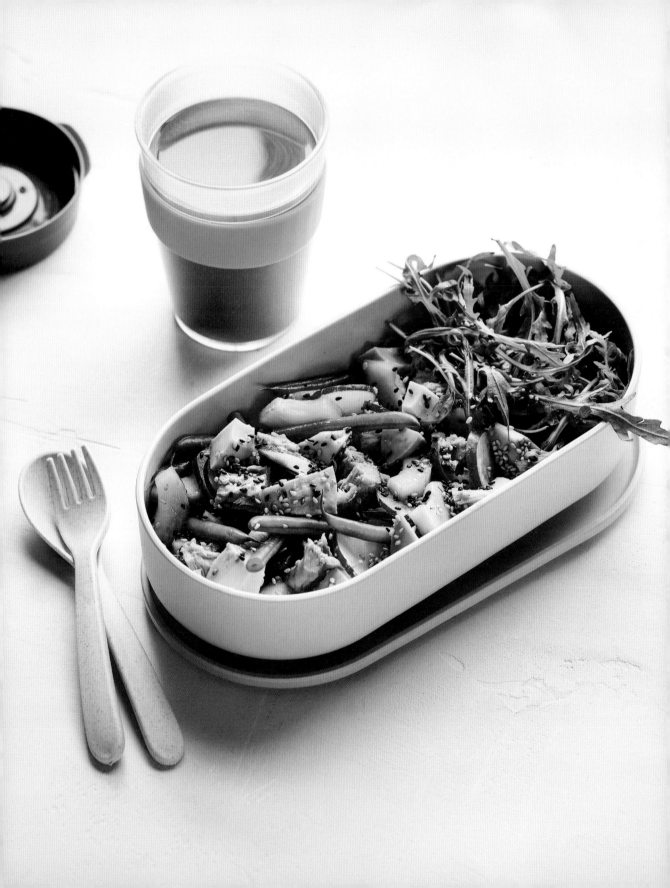

CAFFEINE – FRIEND OR FOE?

A fondness for coffee can feel like another habit you really should quit. But is it really that bad for us? Latest research suggests not, and I've found lots of positive links. Caffeine works as a central nervous system stimulant, so when it reaches your brain it makes you feel alert. For many years it has been used to aid concentration and fight fatigue and even give you the edge in sports (as an ergogenic aid – you'll find it in lots of sports supplements). There is some suggestion that caffeine may have health benefits too, including a potential increase in life expectancy and even helping with some forms of dementia, although more research needs to be carried out to confirm this. Contrary to popular belief, moderate intake doesn't increase the risk of heart disease.

The bottom line is, however, that everyone's response to caffeine is different. If you're sensitive to its effects, you can experience an adrenaline-like response: agitation, sweating, anxiety and even palpitations. It can temporarily raise your blood pressure. If you're reaching for the coffee (or cola, energy drink, tea or chocolate – remember they all contain caffeine too) to get you through a stressful day, it's worth bearing in mind it might be making things worse. If you don't experience this response, by all means order that espresso. It all comes back to balance and knowing what works for *you*.

I have previously been known to drink up to eight cups of coffee a day. But that amount, for me, *did* have a detrimental effect. I thought I needed it to get through my long shifts, but in reality it was making me anxious and agitated and I didn't sleep well once I got off shift. Once I made the link, I started to transition to decaf (if you do it suddenly you can get withdrawal headaches, so I'd recommend swapping in one decaf per day). These days I have one real coffee in the morning, then I either drink tea (which still contains caffeine but significantly less) or decaf coffee. I can't tell the difference and I feel much better.

It's worth mentioning the calorie saving too. My old go-to was a large flat white from a local café. Three of those bad boys a day added up to 1,000 calories! Remember that milk, cream, added sugar, syrups, chocolate sprinkles (just me?) can all turn a drink into the calorific equivalent of a not-so-healthy meal. If your caffeine source of choice is a cola or energy drink, you'll be drinking lots of sugar or artificial sweeteners and other nasties like artificial colours and flavours too.

Green tea, on the other hand, has all the ergogenic effects without the jitters or sugars, thanks to a substance called L-theanine, which is calming. Worth a try?

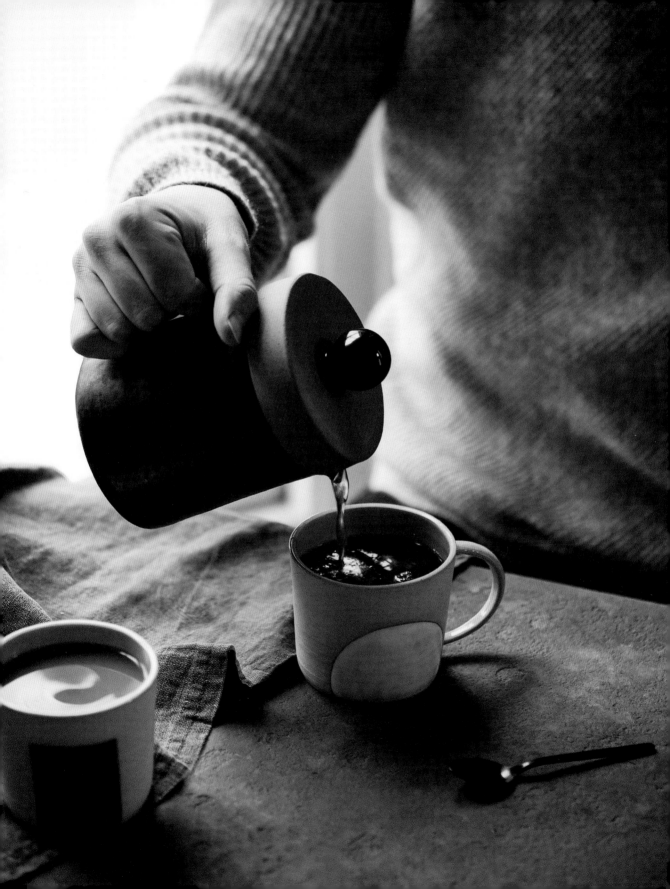

**WHEN IT COMES TO ALCOHOL,
I'M ALL ABOUT BALANCE.**

ALCOHOL – WHAT'S THE REAL DEAL?

Most medical professionals would tell you that the ideal intake of alcohol is none. In fact, NHS guidelines say there's no 'safe' level of drinking, only a 'low-risk' one (which is 14 units or under per week, spread over three days or more).

Me? I enjoy a beer here and there, but I prefer to avoid drinking from Sundays to Thursdays. This creates a structure for my week and means it's much easier to stick within the recommended units. That's not to say I'll binge and have all those units on Friday and Saturday nights – 14 units is an upper limit not a goal. I can't drink the day before a hospital shift either. I don't sleep well after having alcohol and, let's face it, no one performs well on a hangover. I need to bring my A game to A&E and it feels irresponsible to do something that I know would inhibit my potential. Over the years I've also become aware that I feel less motivated to eat well and exercise the day after drinking. I can feel a bit anxious sometimes too. So all in all I prefer my boundaries – a few beers if I fancy them, but not if it's going to have a knock-on effect the next day.

That's just me; I'm not here to tell *you* what to do. Perhaps a glass of wine with an evening meal suits you well. Maybe you're one of an increasing number of people preferring not to drink at all. Or you're aware you drink more than you'd like to or is healthy. Whatever your current situation, if you *do* drink alcohol, I'd encourage you to take a bit of an inventory and look at what, when, how much and why you drink.

THE RISKS OF ALCOHOL

Weight gain

A pint of beer is the calorific equivalent of a packet of crisps or a small chocolate bar, and a glass of wine is only a bit less. You probably wouldn't go to the pub and eat three or four bags of crisps in a row. Think of alcoholic drinks as 'empty calories' (you get no other nourishment from them) and that might help you cut down – and slim down.

Risk taking

It's not just long-term damage to your health that can arise from drinking. I've had patients in A&E who've been victims of assault, theft, had unprotected sex, got themselves into altercations or sustained horrible injuries, sometimes because they've been drunk, lost inhibitions and made poor choices. Sometimes all it takes is one session.

Long-term illness

Regular alcohol consumption – more than the weekly unit recommendation for ten to twenty years – is linked to mouth, throat and breast cancers, heart disease, strokes, liver disease, brain damage and damage to the nervous system.

Poor mental health

There are strong links between alcohol misuse and self-harm and suicide. Alcohol can contribute to, and worsen, depression and anxiety.

KEEP IT IN CHECK

I think alcohol-free days are really important. As is having a glass of water in between drinks. This is not to sober you up – alcohol leaves your system at a rate of one unit per hour and no amount of water, coffee or cold showering can accelerate that metabolism. But drinking water keeps you hydrated (lots of hangover symptoms are due to dehydration), fills you up and slows down your alcohol consumption rate. Try it – it really, really works.

Something else to mention here is the huge range of alcohol-free 'grown-up' drinks available these days. From sophisticated AF 'spirits' for virgin cocktails to AF lagers and beers that look and taste the part, you don't need to feel like you're missing out if you go down the teetotal route sometimes.

There are some super-helpful tools available online to help you look at how much you're drinking, track your intake and, if necessary, cut down. An alcohol-tracking app on your phone (such as the free NHS app Drink Free Days) is an easy way to keep tabs and commit to alcohol-free days.

There's nothing to be ashamed about if you're struggling to cut down on drinking. Talk to someone – a friend, family member, your GP. That first step can be hard, but you deserve to feel better. Help is out there. I've put together a list of really helpful resources at the back of this book (see page 233).

THE BROAD FOOD 'RULES' TO STICK TO

There aren't many food rules that every medical and nutrition expert agrees on. For every study championing one food group or supporting one way of eating, it's not hard to find another saying the complete opposite. So are there *any* consistent views?

Well yes, I've yet to come across any piece of research that says it's *not* better to eat a mainly wholefood and plant-based diet, with low or zero levels of ultra-processed food. In other words, the best thing you can do for your health is to eat real food. I think American writer Michael Pollan put it best when he said, 'Eat food, not too much, mostly plants.'

A plant-based diet doesn't mean being vegan or vegetarian, it means eating natural, plant foods – that's not just leafy stuff, it's wholegrains, fruit, legumes, nuts and seeds as well. You can still eat meat, fish and dairy if you like, but probably in smaller quantities than you do now (which is good for the environment and your bank balance too, so win-win).

As for ultra-processed food, that means fast food, ready meals, highly refined products, such as white bread and white pasta, and products high in sugars or artificial additives, like sweeteners. I think in our heart of hearts we all know what processed foods are. Yes, they're convenient. Often they're really, really tasty. Good for us? Not so much. If you look at the diets and food cultures that keep cropping up in research as healthy, with low disease rates and high longevity, they are all based on real food.

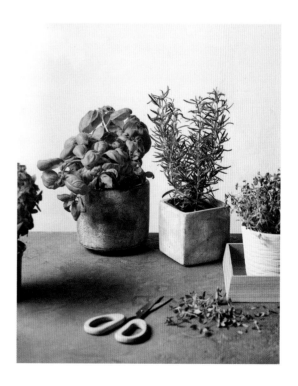

The Mediterranean diet has been strongly linked with reduced mortality and lower rates of chronic disease. If you'd asked me a few years ago, I might have said a 'Med' diet was beer, cocktails and chips on the beach! But I know now it means eating loads of vegetables, wholegrains, olive oil, small amounts of lean meat and oily fish, and lots of nuts and seeds and legumes. It's basically having food as close as possible to its natural state – how us humans are supposed to eat it. Do I eat like this all the time? No, but I do try and stick to that 80:20 rule. Give it a go and see how you feel.

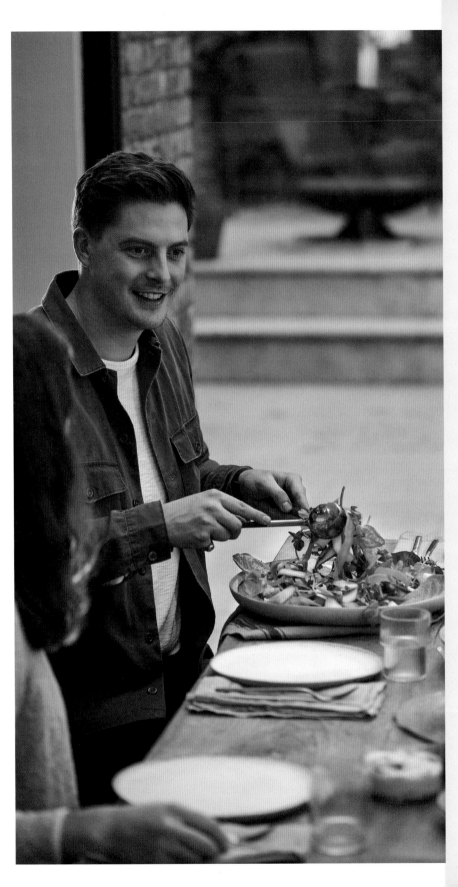

7
mindful eating habits

Stop and sit down to eat
– yes, even for snacks

Put your phone away
at the table – don't
eat distracted

Chew your food properly
– good digestion starts in
the mouth

Put your cutlery down
between mouthfuls –
there are no prizes for
finishing first

Eat with friends/family
– studies link enjoyment
of mealtimes to better
digestion

Make it look nice, even
when it's just you –
appreciate food with
all your senses

Stop when you're full –
eating more slowly puts us
back in touch with hunger
and satiety cues, so we're
less likely to overeat

TRY TO MAKE MEALTIMES A STRESS-FREE, RELAXED ENVIRONMENT.

A QUICK CHAT ABOUT DIGESTION

Good digestion means not experiencing any discomfort like heartburn or reflux, stomach ache or cramps, nausea, excessive bloating or gas, intestinal churning or spasms, constipation or diarrhoea. It also means properly absorbing all the nutrients in the food you eat (and not absorbing toxins your body is meant to expel). That's a lot of work for your body to do, so it's worth giving your digestive system a helping hand.

Digestion doesn't just start in your stomach. It's happening as soon as you put a piece of food in your mouth – before that, even, if you count the fact that how a food looks and smells is already sending signals to your brain to prepare for it. Chewing your food is key because it releases saliva, which contains enzymes that start breaking your food down.

Stress can have an adverse effect on digestion – in short, if you're feeling tense and anxious, your fight-or-flight system will be diverting blood away from your digestive system, making its job harder. Take your time, focus on what you're eating. Doing a mindful breathing exercise before a meal can really help, likewise mindfully focusing on what you're eating – appreciating the look, smell, mouthfeel and taste of every bite.

In short, try not to eat on the hop. I know how hard this is. Life's busy; sometimes it feels like your only window to eat is en route from the bus stop to the train station. But just start trying to slow down, make more of an event of meals. Instead of eating your sandwich at your desk, ask your colleagues to join you in the canteen or outside on a park bench. See what a difference it can make.

LOVE YOUR GUT

You've probably heard of the 'friendly' bacteria that live in your gut. Words like friendly are used because we're used to thinking of microbes like bacteria and viruses as dangerous, infection-causing nasties that need to be eradicated. The vast majority of microbes actually do wonders for our health, so we need to show them some love.

The truth is, we're all walking, talking bacteria colonies. We have 100 trillion microbes living in and on our bodies, they outnumber our own cells by 10:1 and their genes outnumber ours by over 100:1. Most of them live in the large intestine, the lower part of the gut. They're known as your gut microbiota and weigh around 1.3kg! You might also hear the term microbiome, which refers to all their genetic material and capabilities too.

Where do these microbes come from? Well, we pick up our mother's microbiome during birth, we add more through breastfeeding, and our bacteria colony goes on to change and develop throughout our lives, through exposure to dirt, pets and the environment – but mainly as a result of our diet.

And what do they do for us? Where do I start? Your gut bugs help you digest food and extract nutrients from it. They feast on fibre, from plant foods, and as they metabolize it, they release useful substances, including short-chain fatty acids, enzymes and vitamins. Your microbiota train your immune system and produce hormones. They are in communication with many different organs in the body, via pathways including the gut-brain axis, gut-skin axis and gut-immune axis.

There's no doubt this is an exciting emerging area of both nutrition and overall medical research. It's only been just over a decade that scientists have even had the knowledge and technology (rapid gene sequencing) to find all this out. We're learning all the time about different aspects of our health that our microbiota contribute to. I find it all fascinating.

What we know for sure is the more abundant and diverse the range of microbes in your gut, the healthier you're likely to be. Research is still in the early days and it's unlikely to be a cause-and-effect thing, but links have been made between poor gut flora (called dysbiosis) and irritable bowel syndrome (IBS), inflammatory bowel disease (IBD), depression, anxiety, asthma, allergies, cardiovascular disease, colon cancer, Type 2 diabetes, skin conditions like eczema and acne, Parkinson's, Alzheimer's and – interestingly – obesity. A diverse and abundant microbiome, on the other hand, is associated with better health and resilience to infection. It's a very good reason to avoid

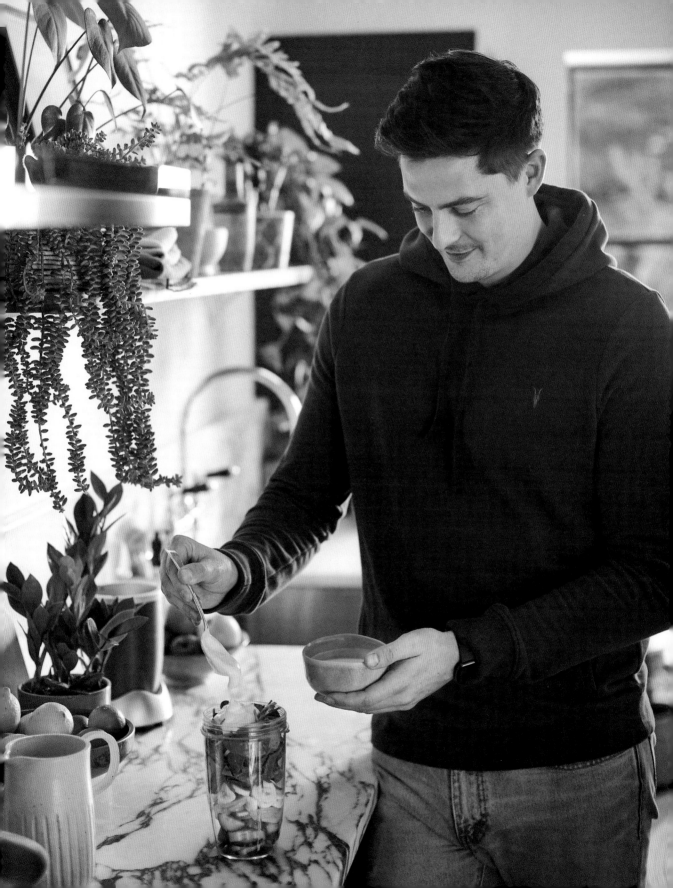

antibiotics unless a doctor insists they're what you need – as they'll wipe out good bacteria in your gut, so you'll need to rebuild it again.

In the future, it's possible that we'll be able to identify which strains of microbe do what in the body – and prescribe them accordingly. We may be able to suggest the foods an individual most needs to change their microbiome for the better. Until then, there's still much we can do. A healthy and abundant microbiome needs a healthy and abundant diet, with lots of different plant foods delivering a tasty range of fibres for your microbes to feast on.

THE GUT-BRAIN AXIS

Can your gut really influence your mental health? The latest research says yes, and it's a two-way street. You probably already agree that your emotions can influence your digestion. Ever got 'butterflies in your tummy' before a date? Felt 'gut-wrenching emotion' after bad news? Then you'll know what I mean.

How does it work the other way around? There have been many instances of people with mental health conditions having gut dysbiosis. And there's evidence that changing the microbiome by diversifying the diet could have a positive effect on symptoms. The well-known SMILES trial found that the Mediterranean diet showed positive results as a treatment for people with depression (alongside medication and psychotherapy). Could it be that this diet reduced depressive symptoms by feeding the gut microbes?

There's clearly a lot of research to be done, but we do know that the microbiome can communicate with the brain via various chemical messengers as well as the vagus nerve, the largest nerve in the body. Again, I think a lot of this we know instinctively. When I'm looking after my wellbeing with a good diet, I feel happier, but when I've had periods of being busy and stressed and perhaps eaten more junk food, it's not been good for my mind.

Food for thought, isn't it?

7
best gut-healthy foods

Vegetables – they're all good; aim to add a new variety each week

Fruit – have whole fruits rather than juice (which removes the fibre and concentrates the sugar)

Wholegrains – don't just stick to wheat and rice; experiment with spelt, quinoa, barley, buckwheat, amaranth, millet...

Nuts and seeds – the perfect filling snacks

Legumes – an underrated, tasty protein source

Yogurt/kefir – rich in important nutrients and packed with protein

Sauerkraut/kimchi – both are an acquired taste but once you get it, you'll be hooked

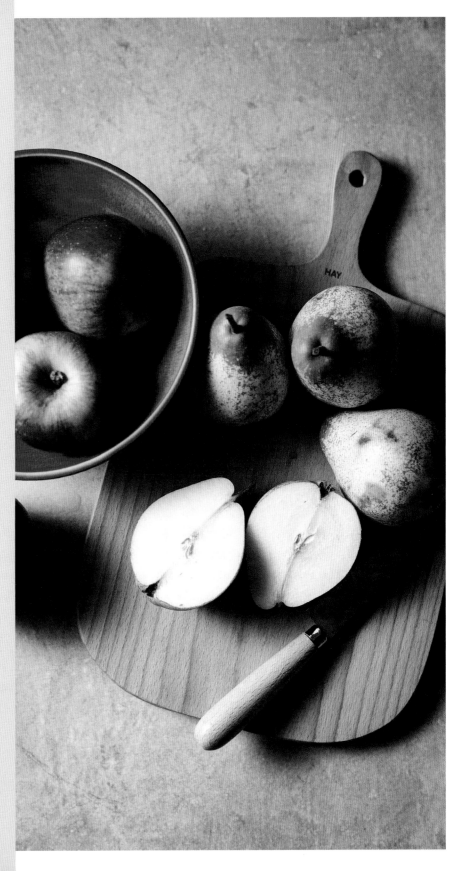

KEEP A FOOD DIARY

I'd really recommend you have a go at tracking your food and drink for a week. It's a great way to get a baseline of what you're actually consuming. Studies consistently show that people tend to underestimate what they eat and drink, so if you're struggling to shift a few kilos, this could be why.

Or maybe you're not concerned about your weight but your health is suffering or you're underperforming in some way. A food diary can reveal patterns you might never have spotted – like the fact you get headaches when you skip lunch, or you snack less when you have protein at breakfast. Increasingly, medical professionals and dietitians are moving towards the idea of personalized nutrition, so here's your chance to get started.

How? You can turn to the food diary page I've included on page 226 for guidance. Some people like to track their food online or use an app (I like MyFitnessPal as it does all the nutrition sums for you).

1. **Keep track of everything you eat and drink. Be honest – it's easy to forget that handful of crisps.**

2. **Take note of portion sizes – we often underestimate how much we consume.**

3. **Keep an eye on the clock. Do you always eat at the same time?**

4. **Pay attention to how you feel before eating. Are you ravenous because you skipped a meal?**

5. **Note what you do while you're eating. Do you look at your phone or focus on your meal?**

6. **Describe your environment. Are you sitting down for a meal with friends or eating on the hop?**

7. **How do you feel after eating?**

It's up to you what detail you want to include and that depends on what you want to find out. All I would say is, be really honest about every morsel that passes your lips. This is about getting a true picture of what you typically consume over a week.

I'm not suggesting you have to keep track like this all the time – that can get obsessive. But if you're looking to get into healthier eating habits, it's a good starting point. I'll do a few days of tracking if I can feel my good intentions slipping. There's something about seeing those unnecessary choices written down that makes it easier to forgo them next time. And I've seen plenty of good evidence that people who self-monitor their food intake are more likely to lose weight if they need to and keep it off. So what do you think? Will you give it a try, just for a week?

EAT PLANT FOODS

Try to eat three more plant foods than you would normally. It could be having a piece of fruit or a handful of nuts as a snack instead of a biscuit. You might want to throw some seeds on your salad, add an extra vegetable to make your dinner more colourful or stir some beans into a soup or stew. Remember — vegetables, fruit, wholegrains, legumes, nuts, seeds (and their oils), herbs and spices — these all count as plant-based foods and they all provide the fibre your gut microbes love.

4

BEING ACTIVE IS VITAL
FOR OUR PHYSICAL AND
MENTAL WELLBEING. FIND
A PATH TO FITNESS THAT
WORKS FOR YOU, AND MAKE
EXERCISE A REGULAR PART
OF YOUR DAILY ROUTINE.

FITNESS & FLEXIBILITY

For me, the definition of being fit is being able to do all the things I want to do, without hindrance. For you, that may be climbing a mountain if you have the inclination and ability or simply walking along a coastal path in Pembrokeshire if that's what makes you feel good. I'm a big fan of going to the gym and cycling. I've also always loved sport and played rugby and tennis at school and university.

I do appreciate though, that for many people sport is not a way into fitness. I know for some it can even put them off. That's why it's important to build a relationship with fitness that works for the individual. The bottom line is, as a doctor I'd just love to see everyone, no matter what age or ability, moving more and realizing how important their fitness is to their overall health and wellbeing, both physical and mental.

I call it functional fitness. It's the kind of fitness I aspire to and the approach to exercise I prescribe when I see my patients. 'Functional' means it allows people to do the things they enjoy – to move with strength and ease. And if they happen to look better in a T-shirt or a pair of jeans as a result? That's a bonus, but it's not the goal.

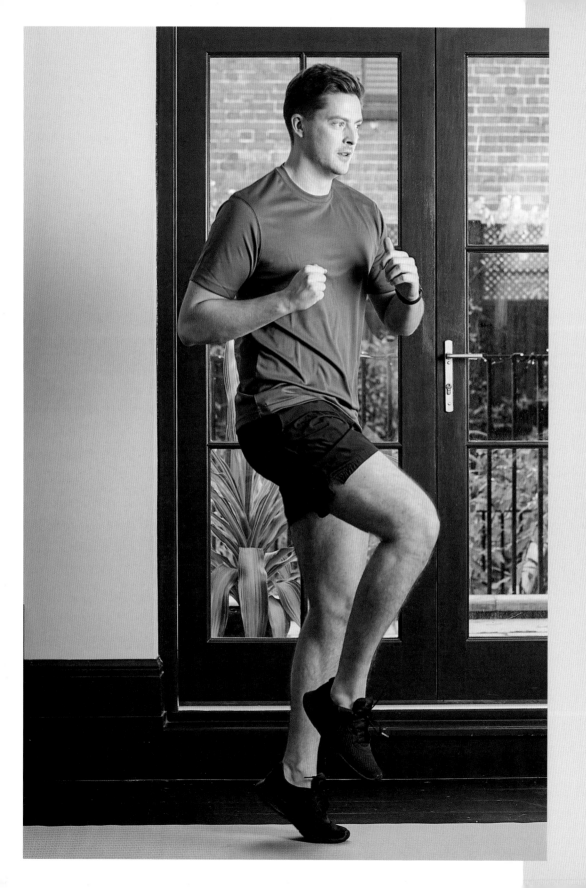

MY EXPERIENCE:
FITNESS IS FOR ALL

Getting and staying fit is something I've been interested in all my life. As I was born in Wales, I'm predisposed to love rugby and, as a teenager, I wanted to play centre or wing. I was tall and skinny and relatively strong, but I was desperate to put some weight on. I was about 14 or 15 when I started to lift heavy weights, probably not with the best technique or form, but I trained hard and used a lot of protein supplementation as well.

On reflection, a lot of it was driven by aesthetics. I didn't like being skinny and wanted to be bigger. I was chasing the wrong kind of end result. Now my goals are more achievable. Yes, I want to be fitter and stronger, but for functional rather than aesthetic reasons.

Being fit is an amazing feeling and it is achievable for the vast majority, if not for everyone. Although I am a medical doctor by trade, recently I completed a Level 3 Personal Training Qualification, the kind you need if you want to work in a gym. Don't worry, I'm not planning on becoming the next Joe Wicks, nor will you see any squat demos on my Insta Stories. I did it simply to better understand the role exercise and fitness play in our health and to be able to provide my patients with the most up-to-date information available.

At med school we're not taught a great deal about the science behind fitness. In A&E we see a lot of sporting injuries, such as sprains and strains, so it's important to know what physiological exercise is beneficial to our patients and what is harmful, as well as understanding the psychological drivers behind their training. It's been fascinating learning how to train safely and effectively, and what happens to our bodies when we do.

When I'm asked about fitness on my socials, the questions are normally about finding the time to exercise and how to motivate oneself rather than the specifics of training. People really do struggle to find ways to fit it in – and if that's you, I totally understand. Later on in this chapter (see page 125), you can find a brief but super-effective workout I've put together to follow when you need to get the most out of a training session. Utilizing high-intensity interval-training techniques (HIIT) and using your own body weight, the workout will raise your heart rate, hit all your major muscle groups and burn calories, all in less than half an hour. But I'm getting ahead of myself. Let's have a look at the reasons why people are struggling to make exercise part of their day – and what we can do about it.

I'VE LEARNED HOW TO GET MORE OUT OF SHORT TRAINING SESSIONS, WHICH IS REALLY USEFUL WHEN YOU GO THROUGH BUSY PERIODS IN YOUR LIFE.

THE PROBLEM: WE'RE SITTING TOO MUCH

Working in A&E, I see a lot of people coming in with issues that are a direct result of ignoring their fitness and not living a healthy lifestyle. And it may surprise you to learn that conditions such as obesity, diabetes and cardiovascular disease are not just confined to older patients. I see a lot of young men and women who suffer from these conditions – yes, including heart attacks. Despite there being an emphasis on men, they are a huge problem in women as well. What all these conditions have in common though, is that they can be the result of a sedentary lifestyle. If you don't move, then the likelihood of developing the above conditions and many more, including back pain, increase exponentially.

So how have we become so sedentary as a society? I think one of the reasons is that many of the people who would be classed as living a sedentary lifestyle don't think they do. The bottom line is, if you're sitting down for six or more hours a day, then you're classed as sedentary. You may not be overweight, you may go to the gym three to five times a week, but if you don't find the time to move regularly during the day, then you could be putting yourself as much at risk from these conditions as people leading far less healthy lives.

In fact, people with a normal body mass index (BMI – see page 111) who are sedentary are potentially at greater risk of cardiovascular disease than those who are overweight and active. It's no surprise that the phrase 'sitting is the new smoking' has been so prevalent in recent years – it really is that serious. A recent study associated a sedentary lifestyle with almost 70,000 deaths a year in the UK and estimates costs to the NHS of around £700 billion annually.

The situation has worsened over the past 12 months, with Covid-19 restrictions forcing people to work from home, not only robbing them of an exercise opportunity during their commute or lunch break, but also reducing the chance for them to get outside at regular points during the day. Think about it. Perhaps you used to walk to the bus stop or cycle to work. Maybe you'd take the stairs six or more times a day, have a walk at lunchtime or go home via the gym. Even the opportunity to move around your workplace to speak to colleagues has disappeared. The need to get up and get moving – preferably outside – is now greater than ever.

CASE STUDY – RACHEL

As a healthcare professional, it's always good to practise what you preach. I see a lot of patients with back pain and what many have in common is they spend their working day sitting down. Rachel was one of them. She had a busy office job and was deskbound; she literally didn't move all day. She was taking a variety of painkillers and having time off work to rest, but this wasn't addressing the root cause of her problem: her core muscles were so weak due to lack of movement they could no longer support her body, particularly when in a fixed sitting position. It was the subsequent pressure this put on her lower back that was causing her pain.

It's something I can relate to: I'm tall and my job can be sedentary at times, but whenever I start getting back pain, I know I need to start moving more. When I do, the pain goes away. I explained to Rachel that her body isn't designed to remain still for that length of time; we are supposed to move. For many years someone with back pain would have been prescribed a month of bed rest, but we now know that's the worst thing you can do. I recommended Rachel continue with her painkillers, but only to enable her to move more. I prescribed a slow build-up of exercise, starting with some of the tips detailed on page 112 and moving on to some light stretching and mobility exercises.

FAT VS FIT

A lot of patients are surprised when I tell them they're better off being slightly overweight and active than skinny and sedentary, particularly in terms of cardiovascular risk. Many point to their BMI as proof that they're fit and healthy, but that number can give people who are sitting too much a false sense of security. They probably don't eat terribly or drink too much alcohol, but if they live in a city, have a job that keeps them behind a desk and haven't exercised or increased their heart rate recently, then they're at risk.

My parents are a good example. My dad is slightly overweight and always has been, but he's strong and very active, whereas my mum is slim but doesn't do much exercise. The heart is a muscle that needs to be exercised so that it can function at its highest capacity. Not keeping fit and allowing your heart to weaken, along with poor diet choices, which damage the vessels that lead to the heart and restrict its supply of vital nutrients and oxygen, can all have detrimental effects. Happily my mum took my advice to heart and signed up for fitness classes and has increased her activity accordingly.

Of course, I see people in A&E who are overweight and also inactive, and are now suffering as a result. They can be massively obese and have knee pain, arthritis and Type 2 diabetes. And the only thing more shocking than the volume of people like this we see, is their age – many of them are a lot younger than you'd expect.

If you're new to regular exercise, do some research into the options near you. Try dance, cycling or lifting weights for strength and stamina, yoga or Pilates for flexibility, and circuit training for getting your heart pumping. Or jog/walk round your local park. Everyone has to start somewhere!

WE CAN ALL BENEFIT FROM MOVING MORE, NOT ONLY FOR OUR PHYSICAL HEALTH BUT FOR OUR MENTAL HEALTH.

FAR-REACHING BENEFITS

• From a physical perspective, exercising increases the blood flow to the brain, which improves clarity of thought and concentration levels. Plus, for most people, exercising keeps them mentally in the present, allowing them to clear their minds.

• Mindfulness is not just about meditation; out running you're vividly aware of what your body is doing, how you're moving and breathing. For people struggling with mental health issues, a few minutes of respite from their crowded thoughts can make a world of difference.

• Being active and exercising more is absolutely key for our wellbeing. This is especially true for people who are stuck living a sedentary life, only going outside to commute on public transport or in a car, and not spending any quality time in nature. I see patients who are inactive and then genuinely feel better if they get outside, if only for a walk.

• If you're going back to exercise after a break (or starting for the first time), you'll see and feel the benefits very quickly. Within a month you can go from walking a mile to running a mile, from performing a kneeling push-up to a full one. So long as you keep changing things up and adding new micro challenges, you'll continue to see results. The fitter you are, the smaller and more difficult improvements are to come by – ask any athlete at the top of their game, trying to get that new personal best.

• Getting outside is good for you. Exposure to sunlight means your body is making vitamin D (which we all need in the UK), as well as providing other feel-good benefits. And if you can get outside in the morning, even better – another recent study also found that exposure to bright morning light correlates with a lower body weight.

• You don't have to spend a fortune on gym membership, fitness gear, trainers or tech (unless you want to). Fitness is free and it gives your mind and body benefits money simply can't buy.

UNDER 18.5
UNDERWEIGHT

18.5 – 24.9
HEALTHY WEIGHT

25 – 29.9
OVERWEIGHT

BMI

OVER 30
OBESE

YOU'RE BETTER OFF BEING SLIGHTLY OVERWEIGHT AND ACTIVE THAN SKINNY AND SEDENTARY.

WHAT'S THE DEAL WITH BMI?

This is a question I get asked a lot. What exactly is body mass index (BMI) – and is it an accurate guide to health? My answer is that it can be a useful tool for most people, if you understand its flaws. This is my quick guide.

BMI is a calculation that uses your height to work out if your weight is healthy. I could show you the sums here, but there are loads of easy BMI calculators online – the NHS website for starters (see Resources, page 233). For most adults, an ideal BMI is in the 18.5 to 24.9 range, while anything over is classed as overweight or obese. But take very muscular people, such as rugby players or bodybuilders. Their BMI might class them as obese even though they're a healthy weight, because muscle is much denser and therefore heavier than fat. That's something that needs to be taken into account when assessing professional athletes – I wouldn't want to tell Welsh rugby captain Alun Wyn Jones that he needs to shift a few kilos!

If you don't fall into the super-athletic category, then BMI can be a useful 'zone' to stay in. But over time you learn what your body's happy weight is. Personally, if I'm sticking to my exercise plan, cycling and lifting weights, then 91kg is about right for me. I'm 6ft 4in (193cm), so that makes my BMI 24.4. When I was on *Love Island* though, the pressure was on to be slimmer and more toned, so I went down to 87kg (BMI 23.3), which was a struggle and not healthy, because I was fighting against my natural state.

As a doctor, I always ask people if they're comfortable with their weight. If they are, even if they're slightly overweight, that could be their happy weight and probably their healthiest. As long as you're active and there are no underlying health issues, being a little overweight isn't necessarily a problem.

SEVEN WAYS TO SNEAK MOVEMENT INTO YOUR DAY

1. Buy a standing desk

Not everyone works in an office, but if you do, put in a request for a standing desk. Not only does standing while you work mean you're constantly shifting and moving position, it also helps prevent the back and shoulder pain associated with being hunched over a computer for eight hours a day. You don't have to stand all day, but a desk like this gives you an option to vary it. So maybe you sit for a task where you need to really focus, but stand for a Zoom call. If you're a freelancer, you can often pick up standing desks cheaply second-hand.

2. Make a rule to move every 60 minutes

If your job requires you to be mainly seated, then set an alarm either on your phone, watch, activity tracker or computer to get up and move around at least every 60 minutes. Whether it's to make a cup of tea or speak to a colleague, moving away from a seated position, if only for a few minutes, is enough to break up a sedentary day.

3. Walk or cycle part of the way to work

A stealthy way of adding movement to your day is by making it part of your commute. Whether you drive to work or take public transport, try cycling or walking instead. If your journey is a long one, maybe park away from your place of work or get off a stop early and walk the rest of the way in. Those extra steps really add up. (Don't do this just on workdays; apply it to days out and weekend shopping trips too.)

4. Take stairs instead of lifts and escalators

Every flight of stairs is an exercise opportunity. Going up and down a couple of flights of steps a couple of times a day gets the heart working, strengthens your legs and burns a few calories, all of which up your fitness levels.

5. Walk when making planned phone calls

If I've got a planned call, I'll do it while walking outside, *West Wing*-style. It's a good example of how to add exercise to a pre-existing habit and will ensure those long phone calls back home or to friends help increase your overall fitness.

6. Build exercise into your social life

Be a bit more adventurous when meeting up with friends. Sure, going to the pub or having dinner is great, but so is going for a run or a cycle together. If that's too much, then go for a walk in a park or out in the countryside. Sign up to try a new fun activity together, such as paddleboarding or Nordic walking. Or resurrect an old activity you all used to do together, like netball or skateboarding – just wear the correct protective equipment if you do the latter, as you don't want to end up in A&E!

7. Wear your running kit when taking the dog for a walk

Super-charging a dog walk is a good way of increasing your heart rate and burning some calories while performing a task you'd have to do anyway. Your dog may need a bit of training to run alongside you, but once they've got it, you'll be bolting your exercise onto a pre-existing habit, which is the best way of making sure you stick to it – see page 118. (No dog? Not a problem! Be a good neighbour and borrow one!)

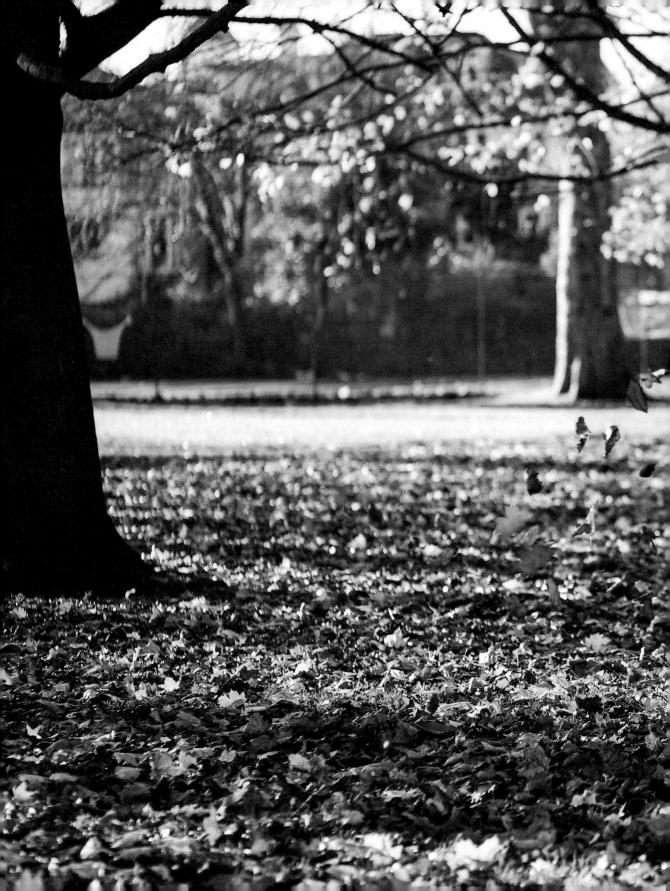

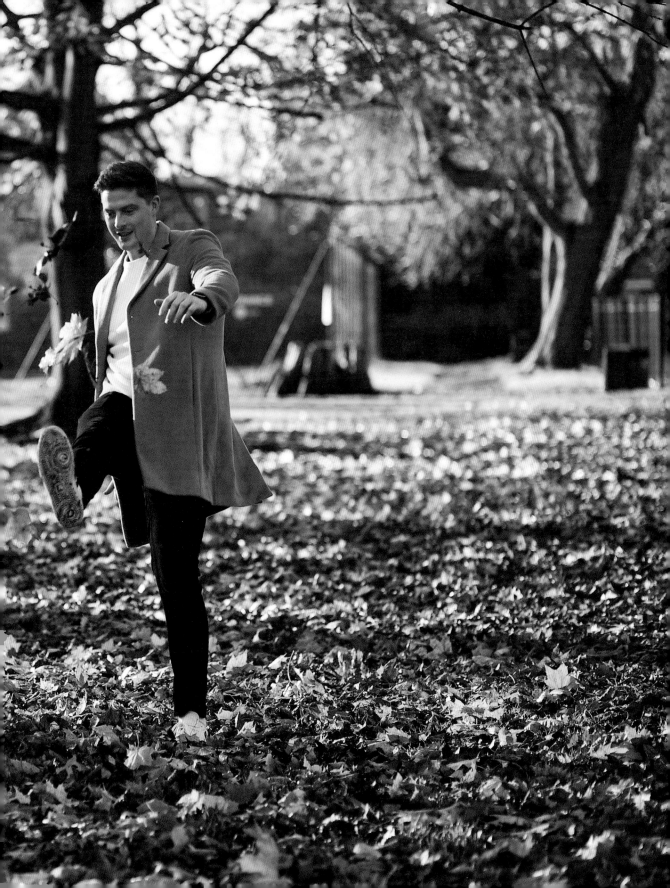

FINDING BALANCE

Hey, I'm well aware there will be lots of you reading this who already fit exercise into their lives – and love it. But, as with all things in life, balance is key. Can you do too much? Absolutely. Part of exercising, in particular strength training, is to break down our body's muscle fibres so they knit back together stronger. Injuries from sport and physical exercise accidents are common, but there have been instances in A&E – albeit rare – of patients who have overexerted themselves to the extent that they have caused damage way beyond what's healthy. And it's not just pulled muscles and back pain.

For a lot of people who want to look a certain way, intense training becomes their life, but I would never advocate going to extremes. Avoiding seeing friends because you're going to the gym instead goes way too far. Check in with yourself and ask, 'Am I enjoying this?' Balance is better – you can always go to the gym tomorrow.

CASE STUDY – PAUL

Paul was an extreme case. This young gentleman came into A&E with extreme muscle pain – he could hardly walk – as well as issues with his urine, which was very, very dark – not a good sign. Blood tests indicated to me he had rhabdomyolysis, a condition that arises when muscle tissue starts to break down and release toxins into the bloodstream, often seen in runners after completing a marathon. I'd never normally see results like that in such a young and fit individual. The levels of toxins in Paul's blood could easily have damaged his kidneys. Some detective work revealed that Paul had previously been extremely fit. He'd just had his first session with a new personal trainer after a two-year break – and had gone into beast mode. I'm just glad he came in when he did, or it could have been much worse. We got him on the road to recovery and he promised to take it much easier for a while.

OK, so Paul was an extreme case, but I use him as a good reminder that it pays to build yourself up gradually when getting back into fitness.

DON'T EXPECT TOO MUCH OF YOURSELF STRAIGHT AWAY; TAKE THE TIME TO BUILD UP AND CONDITION YOUR BODY.

MOTIVATION: HOW TO START

For a lot of people, both those new to training and those finding their way back to fitness after a break, taking that first step can be a real issue. We're conditioned to think that getting fit is hard, that it's going to be painful and difficult. It's good to bear in mind, particularly if you've never done it before, that getting fit can be fun and enjoyable, and the benefits can actually change your life.

I have been fit, unfit and hovering in between my entire life. Sometimes it's hard to see the point in trying to get back to the shape you were in before; sometimes it just seems too much like hard work. But there's always a way back to fitness, you just have to be patient and do it incrementally.

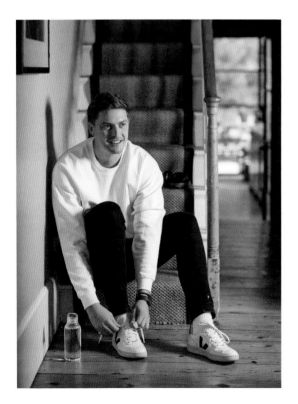

While it's fine to look back at your peak fitness and acknowledge it, your focus should be what your goals are *now*. You may find that you don't want to be back where you were previously or the amount of training required may no longer fit with your current lifestyle. It's simply about finding small steps that set you on the path to being fitter than you are at this moment, a bit fitter this week than you were last.

For some of you, especially if you're new to exercise, those small steps may actually be just going to the gym – not training, but making the journey there and getting used to doing that first. Or if the gym isn't your thing, then just going outside for a walk. See if you can do that three times a week, then increase the distance to half a mile each time, then move up to a slow jog for some of it. I always tell my patients, if you take that first step then the next step will follow.

MAKING HABITS STICK

Your first step is exactly that: a step. It's something that needs to be actively built upon, as you can only rely on willpower for so long. Usually when we make a resolution, we do so at the top of something Dr B J Fogg of Stanford University calls the 'motivation wave'. When we decide to do something at this 'peak', we have to be prepared for the fact our motivation will fall and our instinct will be to go back to the way things were before. So, if exercise didn't have a place in your life before this resolution, you need to address what was stopping you and remove those obstacles. This is why motivation has limited usefulness.

By removing those obstacles you're basically empowering yourself, making it easier to stick to your resolutions. The best thing to do is to make a plan with small achievable goals that help you commit to what is essentially a behaviour change. And the easiest way to make a behaviour change stick, says B J Fogg, is to bolt it on to an existing habit. A habit is an automatic behaviour, like cleaning your teeth or having a shower. You don't question those things or try to avoid them, in fact you probably don't have any real thoughts about those acts at all, you just do them. If you can attach your new pattern of exercising to a pre-existing habit, say, exercising for ten minutes every day before you shower, or using your commute as a fitness opportunity, then it will just become one other thing you automatically do.

REASONS TO EXERCISE: EXTRINSIC VS INTRINSIC

Take a look at how exercise is covered in much of the media and you'll find it linked to fat loss, shifting kilos, slimming down, toning up…you get the picture. While weight management is undeniably a valuable side-effect of being active, when it comes to motivation, it's classed as an *extrinsic* reason for getting more exercise. What I mean by that is your reasons for being active are based on external motivations, with rewards such as a change in the way you look and people's recognition of that, which are not based on the exercise itself.

While there's nothing wrong with extrinsic motivations – I'd be lying if I said my exercise regime is not partially motivated by aesthetics – it would be unwise to use it as your sole reason for training. That leaves you at the mercy of your own self-esteem.

FIND YOUR ROUTE TO FITNESS

I realize I'm fortunate in that I enjoy being active. If that doesn't come so easily for you, don't worry – I have lots of strategies to help. Some people can find the prospect of team sports or physical activity quite triggering, so it's important when finding your route to fitness that you choose something that will work for you. That's not to say that team sports can't be inspiring; for many it's the camaraderie of playing football, basketball or cricket that is the main driver behind their commitment. By having a community around you, you're more likely to stick with whatever it is you're doing.

But if that's not for you, then start with solo pastimes such as running, cycling, swimming (or put them all together as a triathlon). Or you could get your exercise in at a gym, taking a class like yoga or Pilates, or via low-impact activities like walking or hiking, which give you the double whammy of exercise and fresh air.

If you're worried about starting from scratch or returning after a break, there are many initiatives that can help give you that extra impetus to exercise. The NHS Couch to 5K running plan has been incredibly successful in getting people used to exercising again, starting slowly and helping people condition their bodies and minds for running.

If you're looking for a community to inspire your running, then parkrun and GoodGym are great at helping you find a way into exercise alongside others (with the added feel-good incentive of giving back by volunteering).

There's also 'no-exercise' exercise in the form of activities like gardening, DIY or running around playing with younger siblings, nieces/nephews or your own kids – all of those things can be surprisingly exhausting!

If you're a thrill-seeker, getting together with mates and trying a new activity like paddleboarding, surfing or go-karting won't feel like exercise, because it's an adrenaline-filled social outing too. And don't forget dancing – whether you attend an organized class, go out clubbing or have a kitchen disco at home, getting your groove on is probably one of the most enjoyable forms of exercise and definitely the most social.

My point is, there's something for everyone, fitness-wise – you just have to find what makes you tick. Thinking about what you loved doing as a kid can be a good starting point.

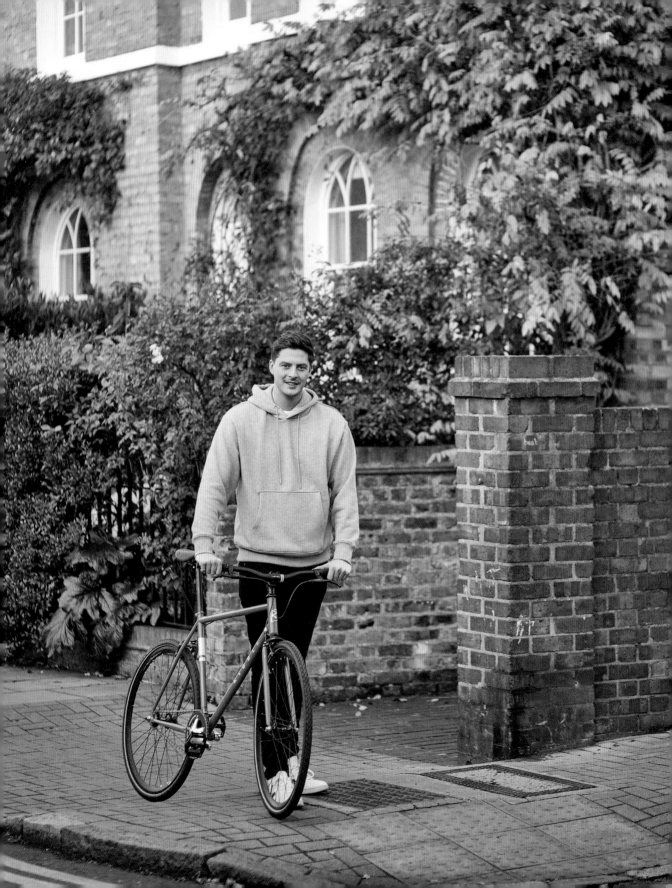

When I went on *Love Island*, I was in the shape of my life, following a super-strict training and food regime. I was lean, with a visible six-pack for the first time ever. But despite what I could see in the mirror, it didn't make me feel good. The drive to maintain that look completely disappeared when I came off the show. Luckily, there are many other really good reasons for exercising. These are known as *intrinsic* motivations and are rewards that benefit you directly, either physically or mentally.

First of all, there's the undeniable effect of endorphins. These 'feel-good' chemicals in the body relieve pain and cause feelings of pleasure, and they're released when you exercise. Endorphins can help you deal with stress and anxiety in the short term, and counter the effects of depression in the long term. Regular exercise can also support your immune system, cardiovascular system, lymphatic system…The list is endless. These are intrinsic reasons for exercising; although you can't see the benefits of doing them, over time you'll feel them. And looking even further ahead, by exercising today you're future-proofing your health for tomorrow. People are living longer, but we need to extend the *quality* of our lives along with the length of them. Here's to enjoying a healthy, active old age!

Regular weight-bearing exercise, such as walking, running, dancing and light-resistance weight training, has been shown to improve bone density in younger people, reducing the possibility of osteoporosis (weak and brittle bones) in later life. Our bone density peaks in

MY WEEK IN FITNESS

I try to get out on the bike two or three times a week for 30–40 minutes if I can. I treat it as 'me' time and get a real endorphin rush from it. I also like to train at the gym two or three times a week and that's enough for me. If I miss a gym session, I don't beat myself up – it happens, it's not the end of the world. Don't overburden yourself with expectations. If you miss one session – or have one unhealthy meal – don't write off the week. Relax, and think of something else you can do that will get you moving. If I'm really busy and I can't fit in a gym session, I'll do my own HIIT workout at home (see page 125). And if I can't even fit that in, then that's OK too. Every day is a new day and with that comes new opportunities to exercise and move.

WHEN IT COMES TO EXERCISE, THE MIND BENEFITS AS WELL AS THE BODY.

our early 30s and the higher the peak at that point, the slower the drop off as we get older (although women will experience a sharp drop off at the menopause). Osteoporosis is something that many people encounter when they're older, sometimes requiring medical treatment. You won't always be able to fix it in your 50s or 60s – it's building up that skeletal muscle mass from a young age that gives you really good bone density, making you less likely to suffer later on. Men have a similar issue with testosterone, in that the level you have in your body drops off as you age. Again, weight and resistance training are essential for maintaining a healthy level of testosterone.

And weight training isn't just for the young either. Above the age of 30, if we're inactive, we can lose three to five per cent of our muscle mass each decade. And between the ages of 50 and 60, muscle power declines by three per cent each year. So, one of the greatest intrinsic motivators for cultivating a strength-training routine, is that it's going to ensure your muscle mass stays with you as you age. You'll be stronger, more agile and look slimmer and more toned – muscles may weigh more, but they take up less space!

The mind benefits as well as the body, as exercise also aids cognitive performance, and there's good evidence to suggest it can help with the prevention of dementia, particularly the vascular kind. It's also known to boost self-esteem, sleep quality and energy, and reduce stress, anxiety and depression. Not bad for a quick workout!

Finally, regular exercise can help you avoid osteoarthritis. Though some people believe exercise can be harmful to joints and can cause wear and tear on cartilage, research shows that exercise can actually strengthen the muscle and tissue surrounding your joints. In fact, it's a lack of exercise that's more likely to exacerbate joint problems, plus you're more likely to develop osteoarthritis if you're overweight and not exercising, rather than a healthy weight and active. As long as you exercise with good technique and the correct shoes for your activity, you'll be doing the best thing for yourself now and for the future, I promise.

THE HEALTH BENEFITS OF BEING ACTIVE

Reduces risk of heart disease, stroke, Type 2 diabetes and some cancers by up to 50 per cent

Lowers risk of early death by 30 per cent

83 per cent reduced risk of osteoporosis

30 per cent reduction in depression risk

Lowers risk of dementia and Alzheimer's by 30 per cent

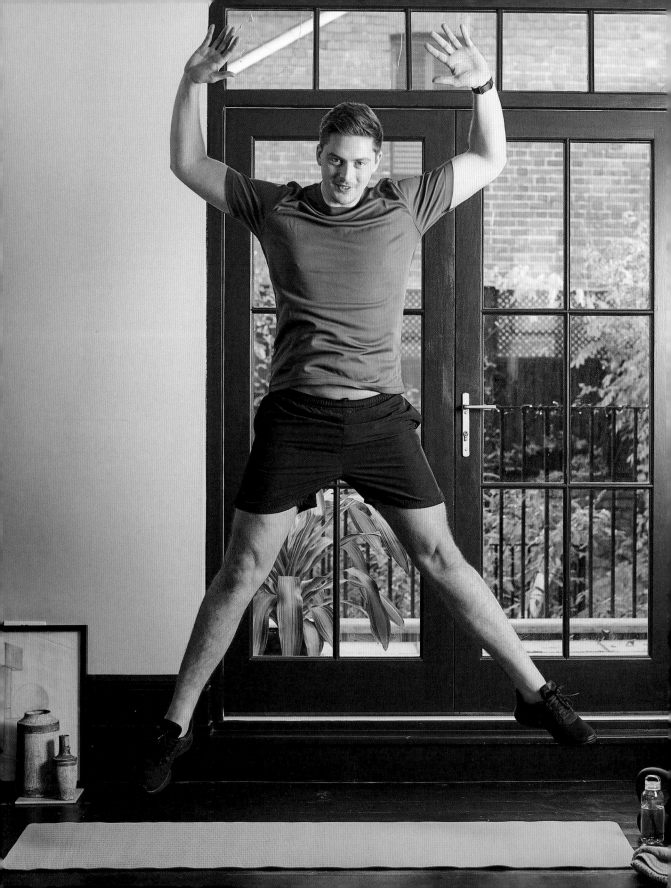

MY EXCUSE-FREE WORKOUT

Efficiency is key to ensuring I stay active and stick to an exercise plan – and I think that might work for you too. My PT training taught me that, by organizing exercises in a circuit and doing each one intensely for a short period, you can fit a full-body workout into a very short space of time. And because you use your own body-weight as resistance, you don't have to use any equipment or go to a gym to do it. You can do the whole thing in the comfort of your own home, garden or local park.

This easy-to-follow, excuse-free, seven-move HIIT circuit will work all your major muscle groups, raise your heart rate and burn calories. If you're new to exercise, try the beginners' variation – they're an easier version. For those with more experience, the advanced option will work you harder.

Follow the exercises in order, working for 30 seconds, then resting for 30 seconds. Once you've completed one circuit, rest for 60 seconds then start again. Three times around will take just 24 minutes!

If you're at a really advanced level, then change the timings so you're working for longer – for example, 40 seconds on with 20 seconds rest, then 45 seconds on with 15 seconds rest. Or ditch the rest time entirely and just work for the full 24 minutes, taking a short breather as and when you need it.

SQUAT

If you spend most of your time sitting down, then a squat is going to be the biggest-benefit-for-least-amount-of-time move for all your lower body muscles. And, if you engage your core, you'll be working on your stability too, which is great for back issues. Stand with your feet shoulder-width apart and, keeping your head up, bend your knees and lower your body to the floor. Go down as far as you can, then push up through your heels, squeezing your glutes, slowly returning to the start position.

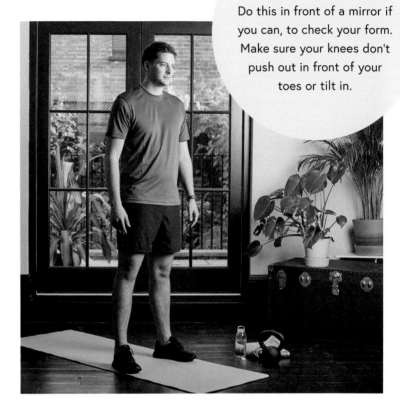

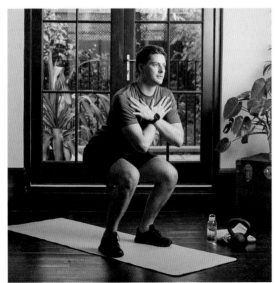

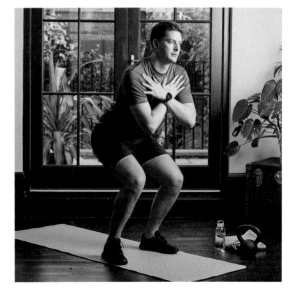

BEGINNER CHAIR SQUAT – stand with your back to a sturdy chair and squat down until you're sitting on it. Rest for a second, then push back to standing.

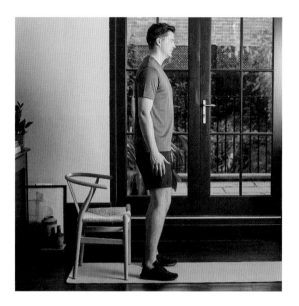 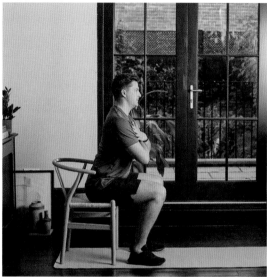

ADVANCED SQUAT PULSE – squat down to the bottom position, pulse a quarter of the way up, squat back down, then push up through your heels to return to the start position. You could build up to holding a weight as you do this.

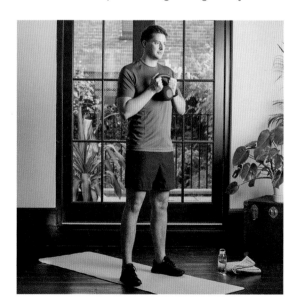 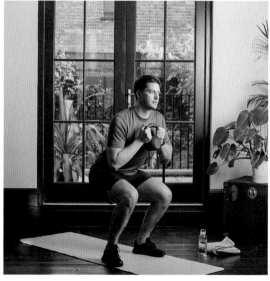

PLANK WITH SHOULDER TAP

Get into a push-up position with your arms straight. Keeping your core tight, touch your left shoulder with your right hand and return to the start position. Then do the same with your left hand and right shoulder. Adding taps to a regular plank is going to work your core a lot harder, as well as strengthening your arms. Repeat as often as you can during the 30 seconds. Keep count of how many you do and then see if you can beat that in the next round.

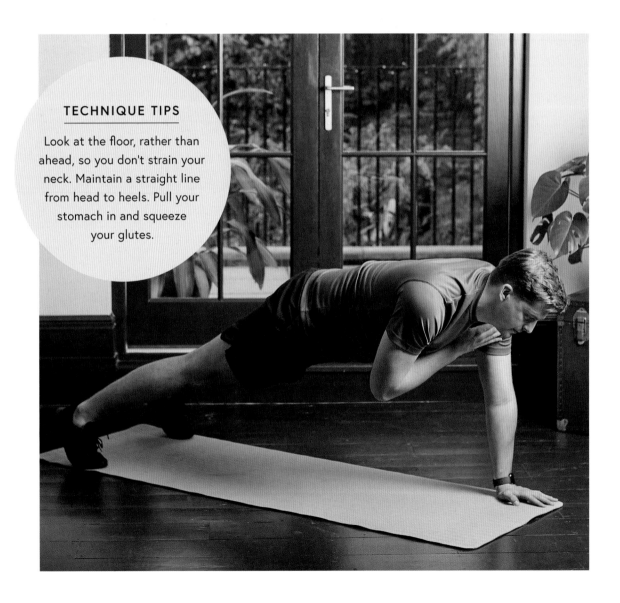

TECHNIQUE TIPS

Look at the floor, rather than ahead, so you don't strain your neck. Maintain a straight line from head to heels. Pull your stomach in and squeeze your glutes.

BEGINNER PLANK –
get into a push-up position and
drop down onto your elbows.
Keeping your core tight, hold
that position for the full 30
seconds (or as long as you can).
Don't forget to breathe, pulling
your stomach in with every
exhalation.

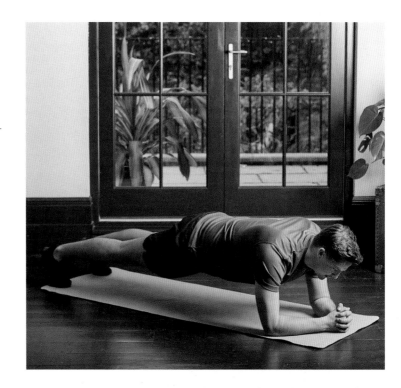

ADVANCED PLANK
PUSH UP – starting in a
push-up position, but on your
elbows, raise yourself up one
arm at a time into a push-up
position, then down again.
Repeat as often as you can
during the 30 seconds.

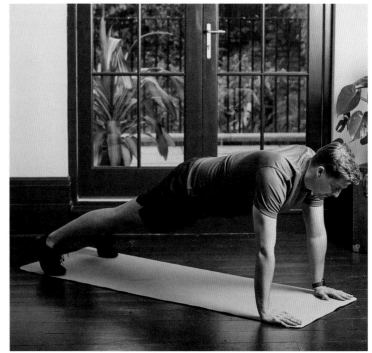

LUNGE

You're working your glutes and the back of your legs here, so it's a nice complement to the squat. Stand tall, with your feet together, and take a step forwards with your left leg. Bend your right knee so it's almost touching the floor. Hold for a second, then power back to the start position. Repeat the move, but stepping forwards with your right leg this time, then alternate for the 30 seconds. Use your arms to balance you.

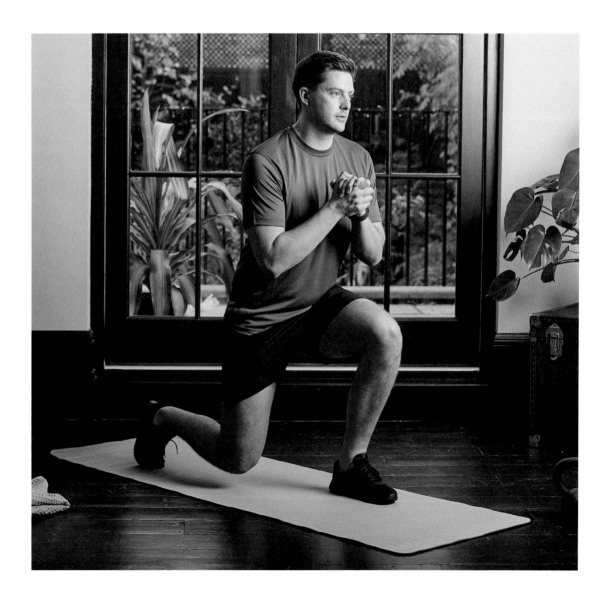

ADVANCED ROTATING LUNGE – when you lunge forwards, add a body rotation towards your leading leg. You could build up to holding a weight as you do this.

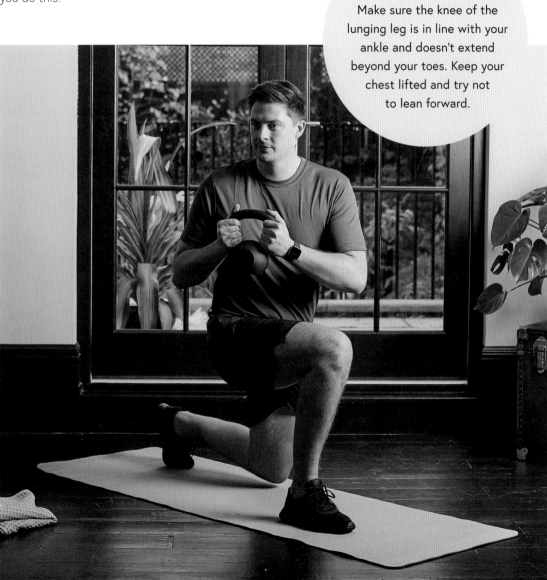

PRESS UP

Back to the floor now for a core/upper body combo. Get into a push-up position, making sure your hands are directly beneath your shoulders. Activate your core and glutes and try not to drop your hips. Lower your chest towards the floor, before pushing back up to the start position on an exhalation.

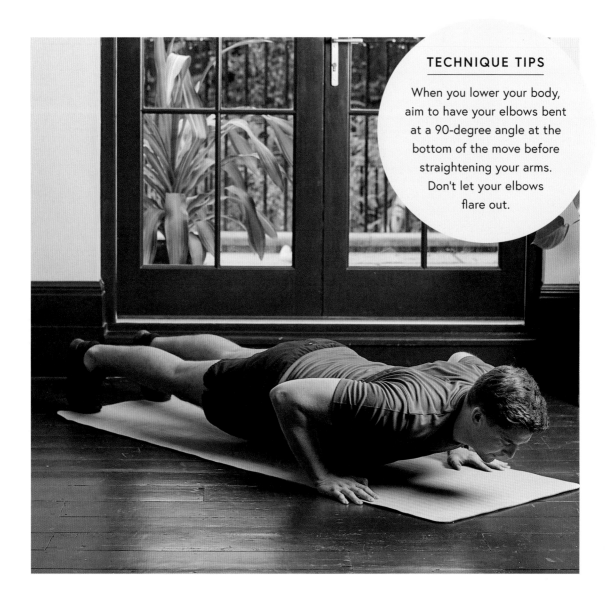

TECHNIQUE TIPS

When you lower your body, aim to have your elbows bent at a 90-degree angle at the bottom of the move before straightening your arms. Don't let your elbows flare out.

BEGINNER KNEELING PRESS UP – start on your hands and knees; this will reduce the amount of weight on your upper body and arms. Make sure you're still aiming your chest, not your forehead, to the floor in between your hands. As you get stronger, you can move your arms gradually forwards into a three-quarter kneel and, eventually, a full press up.

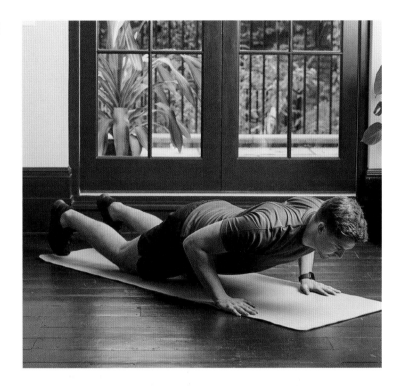

ADVANCED SPIDER-MAN PRESS UP – as you lower your body towards the floor, lift your right foot, bring your leg out sideways and move your knee towards your elbow. Move your leg back, then push up back to the starting position. Repeat, but this time lift your left leg. Alternate between legs for the 30 seconds.

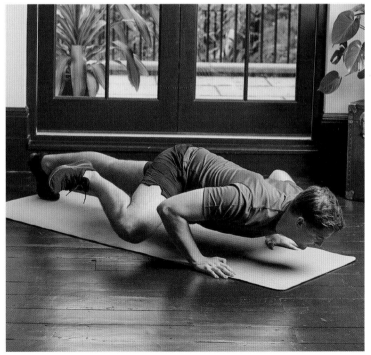

GLUTE HOLD BRIDGE

Lower back and knee issues are often caused by inactive glutes (your buttock muscles). Getting them firing properly will help with everything from walking and core stability to posture. Lie on your back, knees bent, feet near your bum, hip-width apart, and hands palm down on the floor. Push through your heels to raise your hips up into the air. At the top of the move, squeeze your bum hard for one or two seconds to add more tension to the muscles. Relax your bum, then lower back to the starting position.

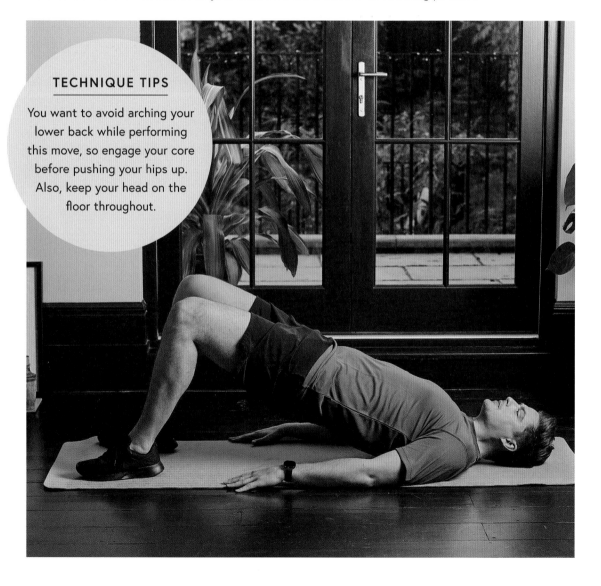

TECHNIQUE TIPS

You want to avoid arching your lower back while performing this move, so engage your core before pushing your hips up. Also, keep your head on the floor throughout.

BEGINNER GLUTE NO-HOLD BRIDGE

— do the same exercise as opposite, minus the 'hold' at the top. Concentrate on curling your pelvis under and lifting up vertebra by vertebra until you get to your upper back/ shoulders, then slowly lower back down.

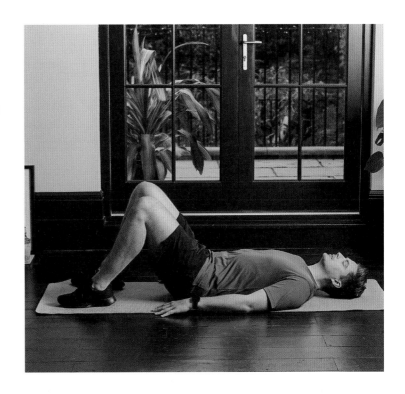

ADVANCED GLUTE HOLD SINGLE-LEG BRIDGE — do the same exercise as opposite, but raise one leg into the air at the top of the move and use a single leg to lower yourself down and back up again. Make sure you do an equal number of lifts for each leg.

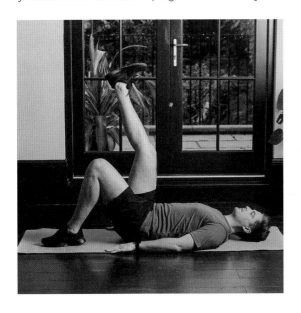
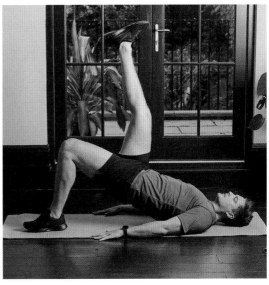

CHAIR DIP WITH STRAIGHT KNEES

This is a fantastic exercise that will work your triceps (the back of your upper arms) and your core. Triceps are quite hard to work in everyday life, so this will give them some welcome stimulus. Sit on the edge of a sturdy chair with your legs straight out in front of you. Grip the front edge of the chair and, with your arms extended, move your torso up and forwards off the chair. Slowly lower your body in front of the chair, hinging at the elbows until your arms are at a 90-degree angle. Exhale as you push yourself back up and repeat. Instead of a chair, you can use any flat surface as long as it's sturdy.

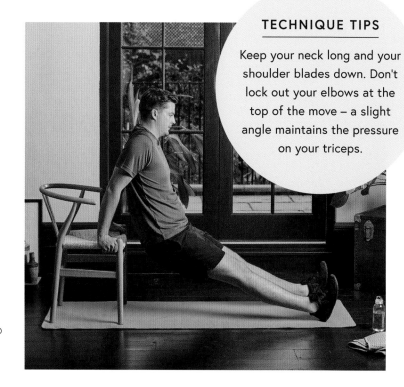

TECHNIQUE TIPS

Keep your neck long and your shoulder blades down. Don't lock out your elbows at the top of the move – a slight angle maintains the pressure on your triceps.

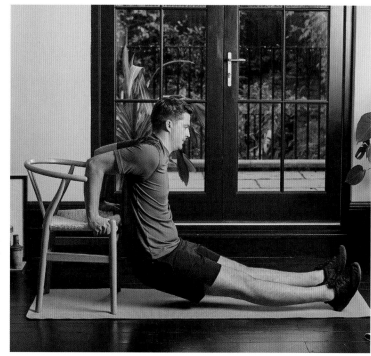

BEGINNER CHAIR DIP WITH BENT KNEES — follow the instructions opposite, but bend your knees and bring your feet a little bit closer to the chair. This will reduce the amount of body-weight you put through your triceps.

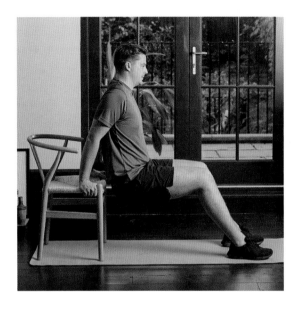
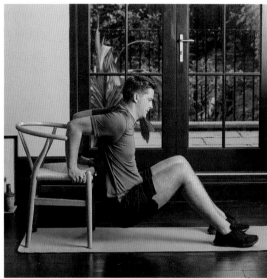

ADVANCED CHAIR DIP WITH RAISED LEG — follow the instructions opposite, but lift one leg off the floor and hold for the duration of the exercise. This will increase the amount of body-weight you put through your triceps.

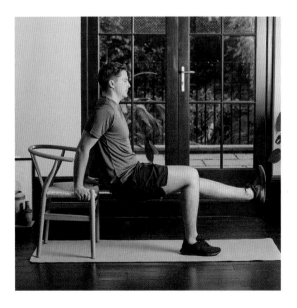
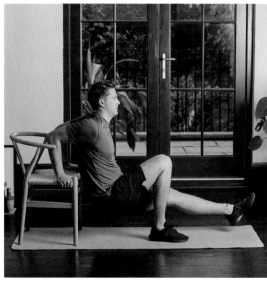

STAR JUMP

A quick calorie-burner to finish up. Everyone knows how to do star jumps and they'll get your heart rate up really high, whatever your level. Stand with your feet together, then jump up, extending your arms and legs into a star shape in the air. Land softly with your feet together and repeat.

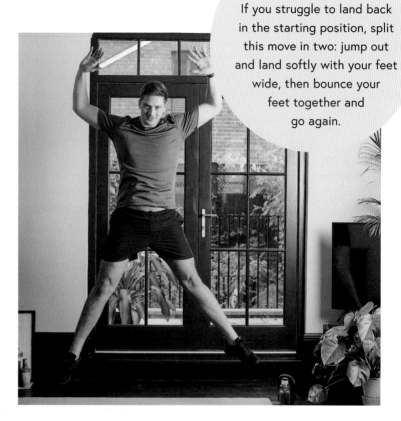

TECHNIQUE TIPS

If you struggle to land back in the starting position, split this move in two: jump out and land softly with your feet wide, then bounce your feet together and go again.

BEGINNER JOG ON THE SPOT — a light jog will get your heart beating a little faster. As this gets easier, lift your knees higher and pump your arms more.

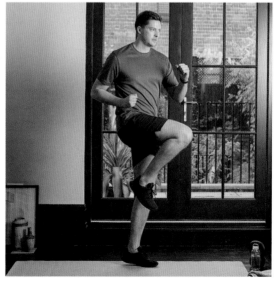

ADVANCED BURPEE – from a standing position, squat down and put your hands on the floor in front of you. Then jump your legs back behind you, do a push up, then jump them back towards your hands. Jump back up to finish.

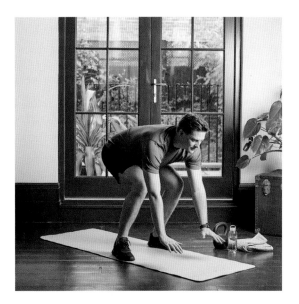

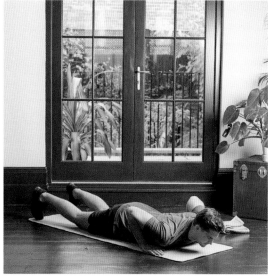

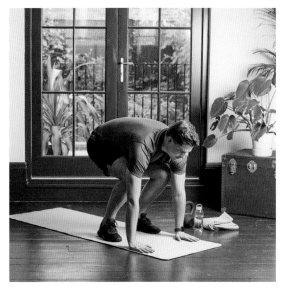

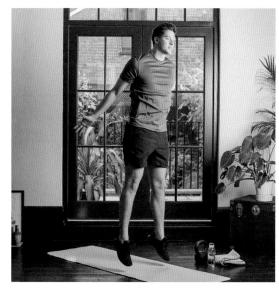

THE IMPORTANCE
OF WARMING DOWN

While you may want to jump straight in the shower after exercising, it pays to spend five minutes cooling down. Not only will stretching out your muscles prevent the dreaded aches and pains known as DOMS (delayed onset muscle soreness), but taking time to wind down after working up a sweat can help ease your body back into its normal state. Remember, post-exercise your heart rate is still high, as is your temperature, and your blood vessels are dilated. Which means you could feel nauseous or light-headed if you don't take time to wait for things to go back to normal.

CHEST STRETCH

This move is good for posture, particularly if you've been sitting at a desk all day. Stand up, or sit upright with your back away from the rest of your chair. With your feet flat on the floor, pull your shoulders back and down and move your arms out to your sides. Then gently push your chest forward and up until you feel a stretch across your chest. Hold for five to ten seconds, then repeat five times.

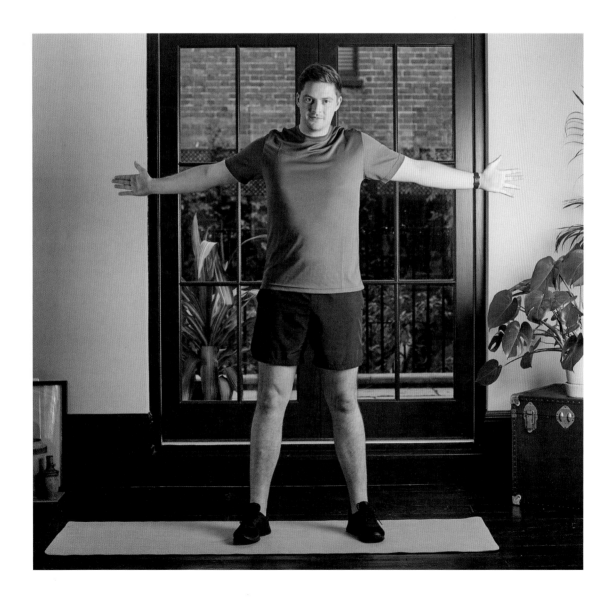

UPPER-BODY TWIST

This will help develop and maintain flexibility in your upper back. Sit upright with your back away from the rest of your chair. With your feet flat on the floor, cross your arms and put each hand on the opposing shoulder. Without moving your lower body, turn your upper body to the right as far as you can. Hold for five seconds, then return to the start and repeat on the other side. Perform five twists on each side.

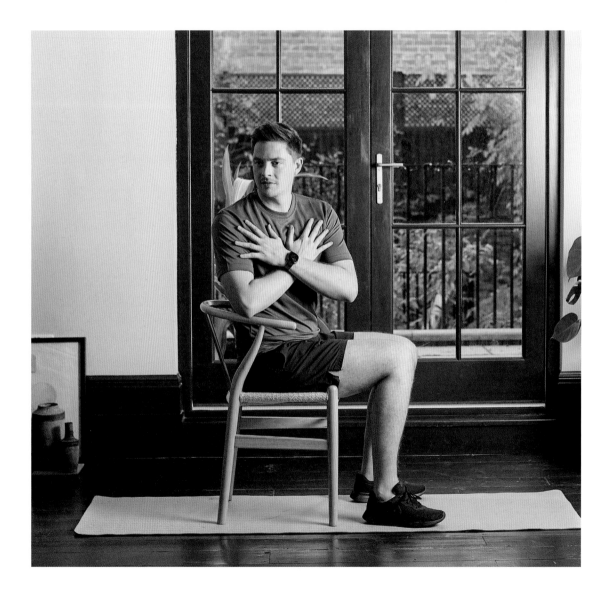

HIP MARCH

If you are suffering from lower back and neck pain, it may well be down to tightness around your hips and thighs brought on by being sedentary for long periods. Stretching out your hip flexors during the day can help relieve this as well as improve general flexibility. Sit upright and, without leaning back, grip the sides of your chair. Keeping a bend in your knee, lift your right leg up as far as you can. Hold for five seconds, then lower it with control. Repeat with the opposite leg. Perform five lifts with each leg.

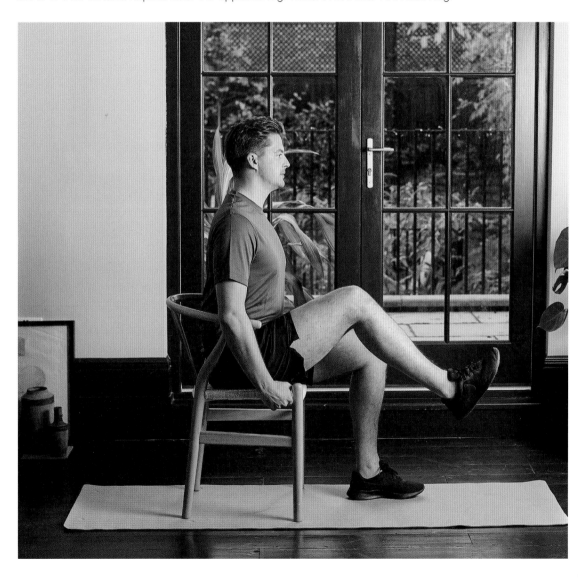

ANKLE STRETCH

Sit upright and, without leaning back, grip the sides of your chair and straighten your right leg. Keeping your left foot on the floor, raise your right leg, point your toes away from you, then point them back towards you. Perform a set of five stretches, then repeat with the opposite leg. Try doing a couple of sets for each foot.

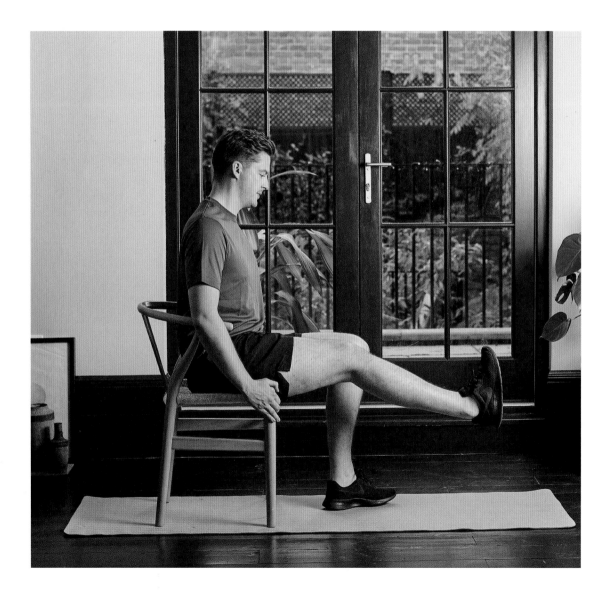

NECK STRETCH

This move is good for loosening your neck muscles if you've been sat at a desk or a counter all day. Sit upright, look straight ahead and hold your left shoulder down with your right hand. Slowly tilt your head to the right while keeping your left shoulder down. Hold the stretch for five seconds, then repeat on the opposite shoulder. Repeat the whole exercise three to five times.

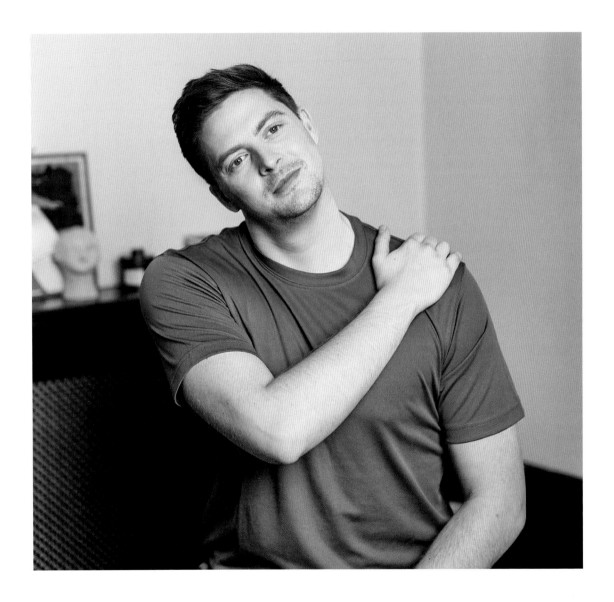

SHOULDER EXTENSION

Being deskbound can cause you to round your shoulders, particularly if your work station isn't set up ergonomically. This stretch helps counteract that. Stand up and link your hands behind your back, with your palms facing down. Push your chest out and, keeping your arms straight, slowly move your hands back and away from your body. If you can only move your arms a little, that's fine; don't force it. Hold for five seconds, then lower your arms. Repeat a couple of times throughout the day.

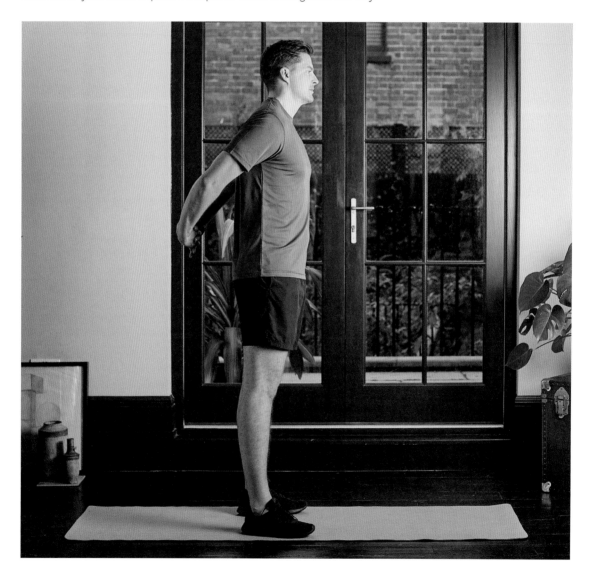

SUPPLEMENTS FOR TRAINING

Over the past decade, a multimillion pound industry has sprung up around sports nutrition. Many products that previously would have been thought for athletes and serious bodybuilders only can now be found easily in gyms, health-food shops and even some supermarkets. Despite these products being commonplace, it's my belief that we should all be able to fulfil our nutritional needs from wholefoods.

In my opinion, it's about what level you're training at. Most people can get the necessary 1.5g of protein per kilo from their normal diet; it's only that small percentage of professional athletes or those people undertaking an endurance event or training at a high level, multiple times a week, who benefit from supplementation.

There's also the issue of quality. When I was buying supplements as a teenager I didn't have much money, so I bought the cheapest products available. As I wanted to gain mass, I was taking lots of bulking powders that were high in carbohydrates. However, when I looked at what was in them, I found it was mainly sugar with a bit of protein thrown in. Not good!

While I would never discourage supplementation completely – I appreciate some people don't have massive appetites and might find it easier to replace a protein-heavy meal with a protein shake – I would advise you to make sure what you take is of really good quality with a decent protein source and complex carbohydrates.

SEVEN TOP FITNESS TIPS

Incorporate fitness into your daily routine

For example, I get my cardiovascular fitness done by cycling to work and taking the stairs rather than lifts when there. These small changes mean that time is not 'lost' doing exercise and it becomes part and parcel of my normal day. You'd be surprised how these short bursts of exercise add up.

Efficiency is key

I enjoy weight lifting and try to go to the gym three to four times a week. To reduce the opportunity of missing a session, I'm a member of a gym that is right next to my workplace. So, in the morning, I cycle straight to the gym, work out for 30 minutes, then shower and change before heading over to the hospital. Not only is it a great start to the day but, because of the location, it's pretty difficult to find an excuse not to go.

Be aware that motivation will fade

Plan for the fact your initial resolution will drop off and find ways to train that don't involve big, unrealistic changes. Start small; micro changes turn into bigger wins over time.

Make things easy

When trying to change a behaviour, every obstacle is a reason to say no to doing it. Write down a list of things that could potentially derail your intentions and think about how you would deal with them before they become an issue.

Look at your routine

When you fall out of love with fitness, you essentially start a new routine that doesn't incorporate what you were doing before, so you need to find a way of reintroducing it into your life. Whether that means getting up earlier or making it part of your commute to work, a new behaviour attached to a pre-existing habit will ensure you continue to do it. As I've already talked about on page 118, if exercising becomes as natural to you as cleaning your teeth or showering, then you'll never question doing it.

Follow inspiring accounts

I find following social media accounts that have a positive message really inspirational. Social media sometimes has a bad rep, but it can be a very powerful tool when it comes to motivation, especially for fitness. I'm not talking about accounts that continually post images of unrealistic aesthetic achievements; I look to accounts that show people following their passion and sharing how it makes them feel. Images of people *being* active, not the results of it. Accounts I follow include Roz Purcell, Shona Vertue, Hazel Wallace, Joe Wicks and the London Muscle guys – their enthusiasm is infectious and, even if you're not doing the same discipline, you can still find inspiration.

Find someone to exercise with

Generally if you buddy up with a like-minded person, you're more likely to exercise. It will also turn training into a social commitment, which means you'll be bolting it onto an existing habit, as discussed above.

HEALTHY TECH

Wearable fitness tech works because it makes you accountable – from a basic pedometer to the highest-spec watch, it gives you that extra incentive to hit your goals, whether you want to reach a certain number of steps a day, lose some weight or improve your sleep.

I use a FitBit, but there are a number of manufacturers out there, the most popular being Apple and Garmin. Products range from simple wristband movement trackers to all-the-bells-and-whistles watches that give you real-time data on your heart rate, calorie burn and pace. I'm all for them: my FitBit supports me in my fitness goals and motivates me to keep moving, even if I don't feel like it.

APPS

It would be great if we could all have a personal trainer to keep us inspired, but luckily there are apps to provide the next best thing. Audio-coaching apps such as PEAR will run you through exercises and routines and basically tell you what to do, while apps such as Nike Training Club, FitOn and Freeletics offer video workouts to follow. Of course there's always YouTube, which hosts thousands of workout videos.

For absolute novices, the massively successful Couch to 5K running programme has its own app that uses behaviour-change science to make the transition from being sedentary to running as painless as possible. And if you're already out there enjoying your exercise of choice, you can track your efforts with apps such as Strava. The free version gives you basic stats so you can monitor your performance but a variety of paid levels up the data and also add an edge of competitiveness with other users if that's a useful motivator for you.

HOME KIT

Having bits of exercise kit at home can really supercharge your workouts. I'm not talking about turning your living room into a gym, but small free weights or kettle bells, which can add resistance to whatever exercises you happen to be doing. You could even make your own by filling empty plastic bottles with handles (like fabric conditioner ones) with sand, rice or water. Even tins from the larder can be used as light weights.

If nothing else though, I recommend getting a fitness mat for training on. Not only will it protect the floor in your home from wear and tear (and sweat), it will give you something to lie on while you do your post-workout stretches.

A word on water

Hydration is an essential part of any diet – our bodies are two-thirds water after all. Even mild dehydration can adversely affect our mood and energy levels. We should aim for six to eight glasses of fluid a day (around 1.5 to 2 litres). That can include tea, coffee, lower-fat milks and no-sugar drinks, but honestly, I'm a big fan of choosing pure water – you can always add a slice of lemon or cucumber for flavour. You'll need more when you're getting a sweat on. But even then I'd steer clear of sports drinks – they tend to be full of sugar and caffeine. For very intense or endurance activities over an hour, an isotonic drink containing electrolytes can be helpful to keep your body's salts and sugars balanced.

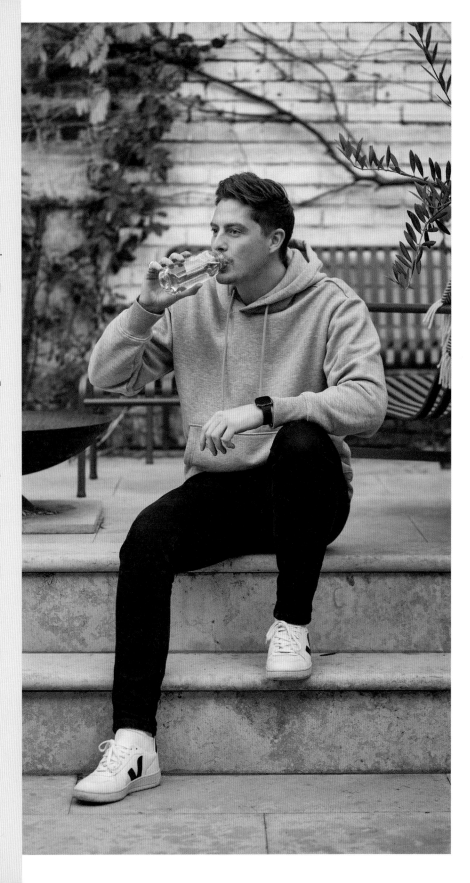

TAKE A MOVEMENT INVENTORY

Being spontaneous with fitness training is great, but if you want to make long-lasting, profound change, then you need a solid plan. It can be really helpful to take an overview of your life to see where you can fit in time to train. Have a look at your week and try to spot opportunities and times when you can incorporate some exercise.

Ask yourself the following questions:

1. Can you do a quick HIIT workout before you shower in the mornings?

2. Can your commute be used as a fitness opportunity?

3. Can you walk some of the way to the shops or to meet friends?

4. Do you need to catch up with a friend on the phone? If so, make that call while going for a walk.

5. Instead of meeting friends for a coffee, can you go for a walk or try a new gym class together?

6. Is there a time in the evening, during your lunch break or at the weekend when you could go for a quick run/do some yoga/ take a fitness class?

7. Can you take the stairs instead of using the lift?

Identify the times when you could work on your fitness, then think about what type of exercise you can do and schedule that in. This is the first step to establishing movement and exercise as part of your everyday routine and becoming something you do naturally.

MOVE NOW!

I'm assuming that you're sitting down to read this, so I'm going to ask you to do something no author wants their readers to do: stop reading. You're at the end of a chapter, so take a break and stand up, reach your arms up to the ceiling and take a few deep breaths. Now walk around – go to the kitchen and make a cup of tea, go outside and get some fresh air. Just stay out of your chair for five minutes. If you do this once every hour, you're well on your way to kicking a sedentary lifestyle into touch. Well done!

5

A GOOD NIGHT'S SLEEP IS THE BEST START TO YOUR DAY – WHEN YOU'RE WELL RESTED, YOUR BODY AND MIND BENEFIT. BUT SLEEP IS NOT THE ONLY WAY YOU CAN GET SOME REST.

RECHARGE

I really hope this chapter helps send you to sleep. Not while you're reading it, of course, but tonight and every night after, because sleep, as I'll explain over the next few pages, is incredibly important. I'd go so far as to say it's like your superpower. A good night's sleep helps your body and mind rest, regenerate and, like the title I've chosen for this chapter, recharge. It helps you be a better version of yourself the next day.

But this chapter is not just about sleep. It's also about being active by day but remembering to build in rest and to not always be 'on'. And it's about recognizing that rest doesn't have to be about sitting down or shutting your eyes either. Sometimes spending time lost in a pastime you love and finding a good 'flow' can be as restful as forty winks. But we'll get on to all that soon.

MY EXPERIENCE: SLEEP THIEF

How do I sleep? Not too bad. I'd probably give myself a seven out of ten on the sleep scale. My main issue is I'm my own sleep thief. I stay up later than I should and I wake and get up earlier than I'd like. So maybe I should have titled this chapter 'do as I say, not as I do'.

I'd say I average six and a half hours shut-eye per night. Although I've got into a pretty good wind-down routine before bed, I'm a night owl. So I'm frequently still up at 12.30am and then it might take me half an hour or so to nod off. The problem is that I tend to wake before my alarm, which is set for 7am. Scientists estimate that we're getting one to two fewer hours in bed a night than we were 60 years ago. We're all different, but I know that on those occasions when I do manage to get to bed earlier, I feel much better the next day. So that's my goal for this chapter: increase my sleep quantity, stop being my own sleep thief.

In the past, there have been times when I've found myself awake at night with anxiety and racing thoughts. I've discovered various solutions to those issues, which I'll share over the next few pages. I've also learned through trial and error how things like my eating patterns, when I exercise, if I drink alcohol and – this was the big one for me – how I time my caffeine intake can impact my sleep quality and therefore my mood, performance and energy the next day.

One of the most important things I've nailed is sticking to regular sleeping and waking times. OK, they can shift to be earlier and later respectively, but I am pretty faithful to those times, whether it's a working day or a day off, and that's something all sleep scientists agree is important. Contrary to popular belief you can't 'catch up' on sleep, so a long lie-in on Sunday morning isn't going to make up for burning the candle at both ends all week.

As a trainee and junior doctor I have done my fair share of night shifts. I used to treat it a bit like jet lag, so if I'd been working all night I would try and stay awake all the next day to get back to a normal schedule. But I'd still feel punch drunk for a day or so. There's good evidence that this disruption to your natural body clock (your circadian rhythms) can have a significant impact on your health, so much so that it's been called a carcinogen.

If shiftwork is a part of your life, I think you need to think even more carefully about a routine that maximizes sleep and rest. If it's not? Try not to put yourself on an artificial night shift by staying up super late! Your body and mind will thank you for it.

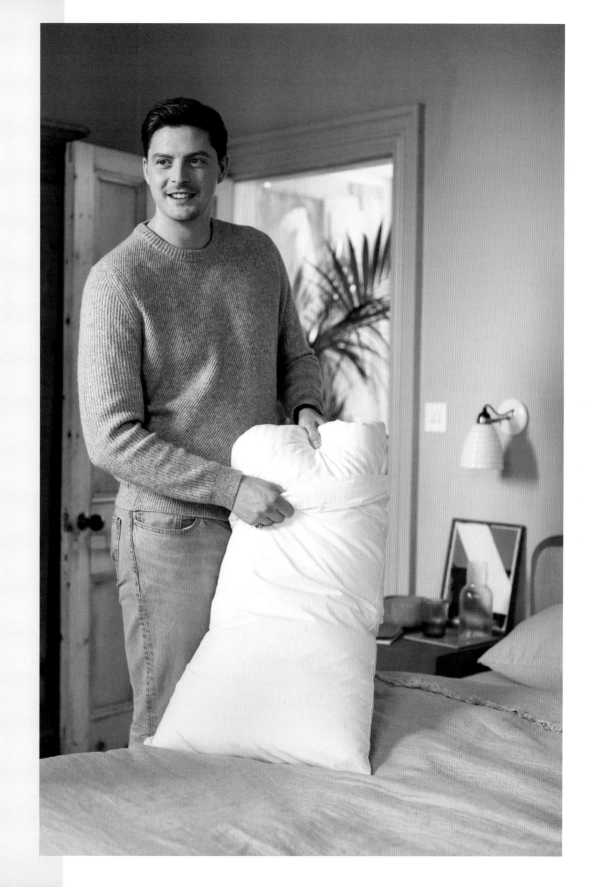

KEY SLEEP FACTS AND FIGURES

We're getting less sleep than ever. According to the Great British Bedtime Report (which was done on behalf of The Sleep Council), nearly three-quarters of us fail to get even seven hours' sleep a night. A third of us sleep poorly most nights. And when asked how that made them feel, over half said their energy levels suffered and their mood was low. Around a third felt their health, work and relationships suffered. If you've ever experienced periods of sleeplessness yourself, you probably know exactly what they're talking about.

Medically speaking, sleeplessness means any time when you want to sleep but can't. So it's not just waking for no reason in the night, it's also being unable to nap in the day if you try to, because your neighbours are playing Taylor Swift at full blast. Or being a new parent and up all night with a baby who doesn't appreciate your need for some shut-eye.

Insomnia, on the other hand, is a more long-term inability to sleep or sleep well, lasting several weeks as a minimum. You may have previously slept well, but go through a period of chronic, debilitating sleeplessness. It's quite a common condition, affecting between 30 and 40 per cent of adults in any one year. Ten per cent of people have ongoing or recurring insomnia. These are the people who sometimes end up in A&E, desperate to sleep – and I really feel for them. It's not pretty.

But whether you have chronic insomnia, occasional sleeplessness or you think you sleep just fine, we could all benefit from looking at our current sleep habits and how we could do better.

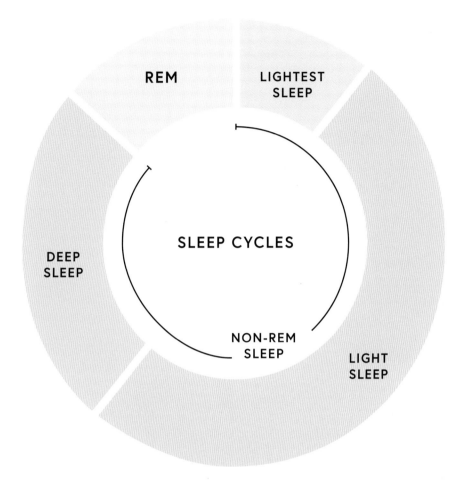

SLEEP CYCLES

Sleep scientists break it down into physiological stages. On average, we clock between six and nine hours of sleep at night, in four or five separate cycles, each lasting roughly 90 minutes. You wake up briefly between most cycles but don't tend to remember. Each of these cycles then has five stages: drowsiness, light sleep, two stages of deep sleep and REM sleep. A healthy adult's sleep comprises around 25 per cent deep sleep, 50 per cent light sleep and 25 per cent REM (when you do most of your dreaming).

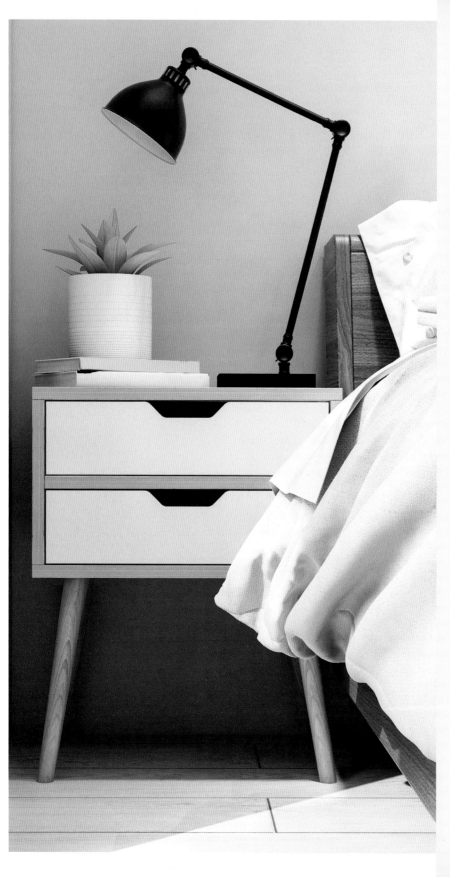

7
signs you're not getting enough sleep

You rarely clock more than six hours a night

You don't go to bed when you feel tired, but when you've finished everything you want or have to do

You have trouble dropping off or you're asleep the second you lie down

You can't sleep without alcohol, or prescription or recreational drugs

You often wake during the night or before your alarm and can't get back to sleep

You curse your alarm and take forever to feel awake

You feel exhausted during the day and can't cope without caffeine

WHY SLEEP MATTERS

These days we wear our busy lives as a badge of honour. We might not have been socializing as much recently thanks to the pandemic, but for lots of us working at home has meant longer hours than ever – and staying up late to reclaim some 'me time'. There's still a funny idea equating long hours of work with success and achievement. And I hate the phrase 'I'll sleep when I'm dead' because, in actual fact, lack of sleep will rob years from your life.

Sleep is a restorative process for both body and mind. There is not an organ in the body that doesn't benefit. It enhances brain function – processing and learning from what's happened that day, boosting memory, logic, decision-making and creativity. Sleep reboots our immunity and metabolism and gives our gut microbes a chance to replenish themselves (for why this is important, see page 96). It lowers blood pressure and helps protect our heart. Every single cell benefits as, overnight, your body goes through a necessary growth and repair process that's been likened to spring-cleaning.

On a daily basis, sleeping well means you're more likely to make healthy food choices the next day – while sleeping less suppresses a hormone that controls appetite, so you'll probably eat more, and less healthily. Sleeping well makes you less likely to reach for caffeine and sugar to power you through. And you'll feel more energized and motivated to exercise.

Over time, poor-quality sleep and sleep deprivation increase your risk of being overweight or obese, and developing depression and anxiety. Sleeping badly can suppress your immunity and make you more likely to get ill. It can disrupt blood sugar to levels that would be classed as pre-diabetic. It's even linked with a range of serious conditions associated with ageing, such as Type 2 diabetes, cardiovascular disease and dementia.

I learned a lot of this from the neuroscientist Matthew Walker, whose book *Why We Sleep* is mind-blowing (see Resources, page 233, or check out some of the podcasts he's appeared on). Matthew points out that humans are the only species that deliberately deprive themselves of sleep with no legitimate gain. Crazy, isn't it?

SLEEP HYGIENE

I really like this term for describing the basic rules we can put in place to sleep better every night. Don't worry, it's got nothing to do with hand sanitizer or masks (well, except maybe eye masks). It's about creating the environment and routine that, experts know, give you the best chance of falling asleep and having good-quality rest. Below is a list of suggestions I've picked up from sleep scientists, reading around the topic, and from my own trial and error. Even if you think you sleep well enough already, pick a few of them to try out and see what difference they can make.

YOUR BEDROOM

- Is your bedroom a nice, calm, welcoming place to be? Could you invest a little time, money or creativity into making it more of a sanctuary? Think cosy blankets and fairy lights. I'm a fan of houseplants too, and they're not only soothing to look at, they help clean the air as well.

- A decent bed is pretty important. How old is your mattress? Is it comfortable? Big enough? If you can't afford a new one, things like mattress toppers and new pillows can make a real difference to your posture as you sleep, relieving back and neck aches.

- How dark is it? When it's dark, our brains release the hormone melatonin from the pineal gland and this makes us sleepy. There's evidence to suggest even a small amount of light can disrupt this natural process and impact how deep into sleep you go. It's not always easy to shut all the light out, especially if you live in a city. Blackout blinds are great, as is making sure there are no lights in the room from tech (more to come on this). But if you can't get complete darkness, think about trying an eye mask.

- The same goes for noise – we can't necessarily control how loud our flatmates, the family or the neighbour's TV are. But we can wear earplugs. I find the foam ones comfortable and effective.

LIKE MOST ANIMALS, HUMANS ARE HARD-WIRED TO SLEEP AT DUSK AND WAKE AT DAWN.

- How hot is it? It sounds counterintuitive when you think of how a hot, stuffy room makes you feel sleepy, but it's actually much better for you and more conducive to sleep if the room is cooler. According to The Sleep Council, body heat peaks in the evening, then drops to its lowest levels when we're asleep, so the optimum bedroom temperature is 16–18°C. I always make sure the heating goes off before bed. Having a window open a little, even in winter, is good too – fresh air means I wake feeling clear-headed. When it's cooler, your extremities cool down first, so it's good to keep your hands and feet warm to make sure that doesn't keep you awake. Thus it's a yes for the fleecy bedsocks, but ditch the onesie.

- Do you share a bed? Nice as it is to be intimate with someone else, it's hard to tailor such an individual thing as sleep when so many of the variables have to match both your requirements. One simple hack is to do as the Europeans do and share one bed, but have two single duvets. No fights about who's hogging the covers and you can each regulate your own temperature.

Research by Oxford Economics found sleep has more influence over our health and happiness than income, exercise, sex life and social connections. It found a good night's sleep was equal to having four times our salary in terms of boosted mood.[2]

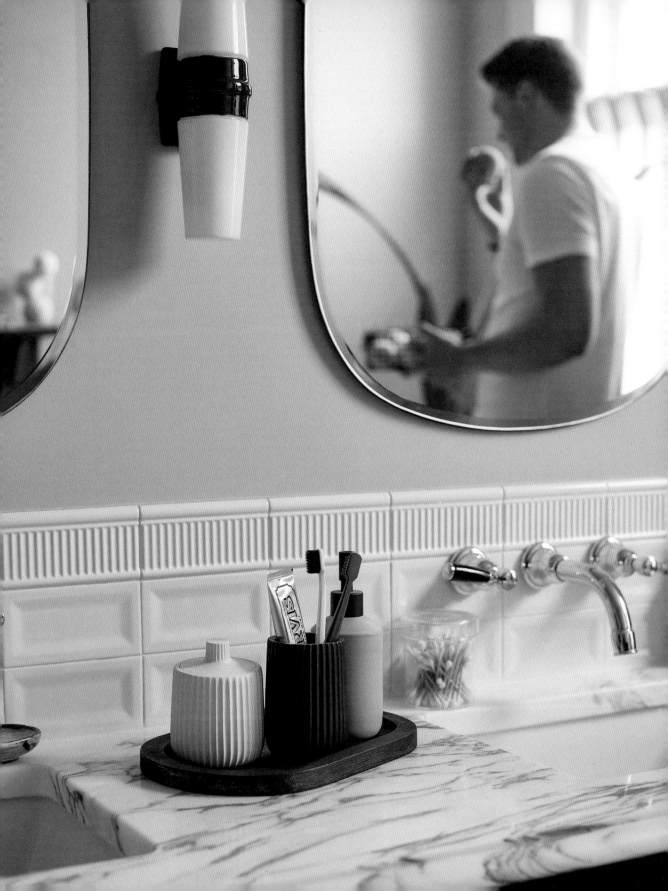

YOUR ROUTINE

- All the evidence points to the importance of going to bed and getting up at roughly the same time each day. Yes, even at weekends. It's much better for your biological clock. OK, we all have late nights sometimes, and lazy mornings in bed can be bliss. But wake up and read the papers, don't slumber on.

- Weird as it sounds, sleeping better starts the minute you wake up. Daylight is your friend, so open the curtains and let it in when you get up. Go outside as soon as possible. Not only does it make you feel more 'with it', it keeps your circadian rhythms on track.

- If you can get out and exercise early – cycling to work or going for a pre-work run if you work from home – that will really help. In order to sleep well, you need to tire yourself out enough during the day. It explains that vicious cycle of a sedentary job that makes you feel lethargic, so your metabolism slows, so you don't get such good sleep despite feeling knackered, then you wake even more groggy. Research, and common sense, say exercise will promote better sleep. So get moving!

- In the evenings, dim the lights (I'm a big fan of scented candles for a relaxing vibe). The last thing a sleepless brain needs is to be stimulated by bright, artificial lights. They will just suppress the melatonin that triggers all those restorative processes in the body.

- Find a wind-down routine that suits you. It might be a bit of TV or a podcast, listening to music or having a bath. (Side note: I always find it problematic that the news is on so late at night. National and global politics and bedtime don't mix, so I get my news fix during the day and save evening TV for Netflix fun.)

- If you like to read a good novel in bed, keep it up. Scientists say that by actively engaging your imagination, reading can put your mind into an altered state of consciousness, preparing it for sleep. Plus, a University of Sussex study found just six minutes of reading reduced stress levels by 68 per cent.[3]

- There are some great relaxing yoga routines you can follow on YouTube. I'm not a yogi myself, but I'm told poses involving forward bends are sleep promoting. What I would caution against though is doing more vigorous exercise late in the evening. Fine if you hit the gym after work, but I wouldn't do anything too active within two hours of going to bed, as it takes too long for your heart rate and temperature to come down – so you'll still be a bit wired come bedtime, even though you might feel shattered!

FOOD AND DRINK

- I write about alcohol and caffeine in more detail in Chapter 3. Suffice to say here that neither is going to help your sleep. Alcohol is a sedative, so it might send you off into a sleep-like state (which explains the term 'nightcap'), but it prevents good-quality sleep. You don't reach the deeper states of sleep, so you often wake in the night or just feel plain exhausted the next day. I know *I* experience this after anything more than a couple of beers or glasses of wine. Neuroscientist Matthew Walker has fascinating insights on this topic (see Resources, page 233), explaining why you can have crazy dreams in the night following a boozy evening (it's your brain trying to get more REM sleep).

- Caffeine is a stimulant so it's clearly going to interfere with sleep in a more obvious way. It can take eight hours to wear off. Everyone's tolerance is different, but as a rule avoiding caffeine in the evening is wise. For some of us, even earlier is a better idea. I used to mainline flat whites all day and wonder why I felt wired when I got home. I used to drink tea right up to bedtime too. Since I've switched to decaf once I've had my morning coffee and a couple of teas, I sleep much better. Don't forget it's in cola, energy drinks, green tea and chocolate too, as well as lots of fitness supplements and shakes.

- OK, it's not a food, but nicotine also interferes with sleep – because it's a stimulant and also because you might wake early due to withdrawal symptoms.

- With food, I think it's a case of trial and error. No one wants to lie down after a big meal and intuitively it doesn't make much sense to go to bed soon after eating. Hence the advice is normally to leave two to three hours between your evening meal and bedtime. I'd leave it even longer after rich or spicy meals or you'll be kept awake with indigestion or heartburn. All that said, there's no point going to bed hungry either. If you ate early and feel peckish later in the evening, then a small snack is fine. After speaking to dietitian friends, I'd advise going with some sort of slow-release carb and protein combo, like an oatcake with nut butter. Avoid too much sugar or dark chocolate (which contains caffeine). You may read all sorts of things about foods like lettuce or turkey or bananas helping with sleep, thanks to certain chemicals they contain. I can't find any evidence they contain enough to make a difference, but if you want a pre-bed banana or turkey sandwich then, hell, who am I to stop you?

THE GREAT TECH TURN-OFF

Minimize screen time in the evenings – this is simply one of the most important things you can do to help your sleep. It's another one of those 'do as I say, not as I do' moments, because I'm guilty of staying on my phone too late. I am trying to stop!

So why does it matter? Your phone, tablet, laptop, games console and TV all emit blue light and this is known to suppress production of melatonin, so it's switching off that signal that tells your brain it's time to sleep. There have been countless studies to show that, even if you still get to sleep fine, it's probably not restful sleep – you don't spend long enough in each sleep stage and scans have shown altered brain waves that adversely affect sleep.

Try to come off your tech for at least 90 minutes before going to bed. If that's too hard, start with five minutes and add another five each day. TV is not so bad, as you sit further away from it. And original Kindles are blue-light free. But e-readers like Kindle Fire aren't, and reading a book on your laptop is not good either.

Have a 'no tech in the bedroom' rule. There are a few exceptions (see page 172), but I do think this is a really good habit to get into.

A NOTE ABOUT BATH BOMBS

If you follow me on Instagram, then you'll already know about my obsession with bath bombs. Throwing one into a hot bath and watching it fizz around and turn the water multicoloured is a definite relaxing pre-bed ritual for me. I highly recommend it!

Baths in general are really beneficial at night and it's all down to the temperature change being a stimulus for sleep. Sinking into the warm water brings blood to the surface of your body, gently raising your overall body temperature. Then, when you step out, your core temperature starts to drop and this triggers your sleep mechanism.

If bath bombs aren't your thing, try adding Epsom salts or magnesium flakes. The mineral magnesium is a natural relaxant that's absorbed well through the skin. It's particularly good after exercise or illness, if you have aches and pains, and can help ease cramps. And if you suffer from restless legs that keep you awake at night, magnesium is also thought to help with this.

WHAT TO DO IF YOU CAN'T SLEEP

If you're waking regularly because you need a wee, or it's too hot or too cold, or your partner is snoring, or for any other reason that you can control, then take action. Stop drinking so much herbal tea before bed, turn the heating off, buy those earplugs...

But what if you wake for seemingly no reason and can't get back to sleep? Whatever you do, don't just lie there worrying about the fact you're not asleep. I know what it's like – I've had times in my life when that's been me, every night. It's especially common when you're stressed – you wake and anxious thoughts just flood your head.

What works for me (and the experts I asked all agreed) is to get up. I'll walk around, maybe have a small glass of water or a camomile tea. I might read for a bit – but a book or magazine, nothing online, and I resist the urge to check my phone or watch TV. Then I'll go back to bed when I actually feel I'm nodding off.

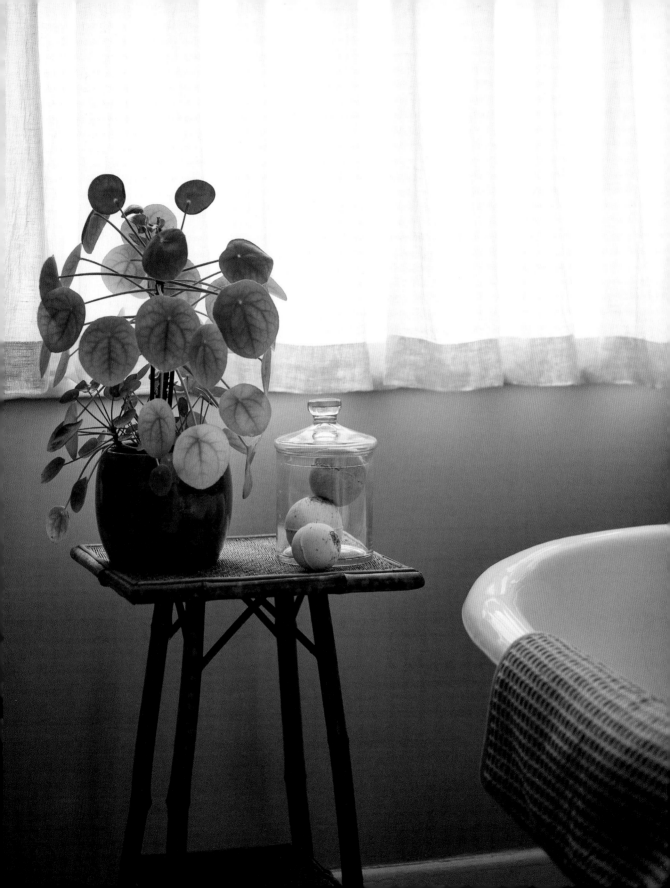

TRY AND HAVE A DEFAULT ROUTINE – EVEN IF YOUR EARLY START MEANS YOU TAKE THE ODD AFTERNOON POWER NAP.

Breathing exercises can be good to get your mind out of an alert, anxiety state. There are so many different techniques to look up and try. I'd simply suggest breathing in and out deeply and slowly through your nose for the count of four, pausing in between each in and out breath. Visualization is another popular technique, although it's not something I've tried. Whether it's counting sheep, imagining yourself floating on a cloud or picturing each muscle of your body becoming soft and heavy, see what might work to help you.

TO NAP...OR NOT TO NAP?

Not everyone can nap. It's a skill I've always struggled with and I find if I do nod off I stay asleep too long, then feel groggy. But others swear by it and apparently it's a skill that can be learned. One NASA study on pilots found their performance and alertness improved after a 26-minute mid-flight nap – don't worry, they got co-pilots to take over! And neuroscientists say we're actually programmed to need two sleeps a day – so southern Europeans have got it right with their siestas. Depending on when you get up, about mid-way through your day is the best time to sneak off to the staff room for a doze.

Sleep experts agree that the ideal nap length is either ten to twenty minutes (so you don't go into deep sleep) or, if you have time, ninety minutes to two hours (so you go through a whole sleep cycle). Either way, if you set an alarm, you should wake during a light sleep phase and therefore not feel that grogginess – which, by the way, is called 'sleep inertia'.

If you suffer from insomnia though, they suggest you try not to nap during the day, much as you might feel compelled to – as that could add to your difficulty sleeping that night, which makes sense.

WHY REST MATTERS

It's not ideal to be on the go all day, then crashed out at night. Or to be sedentary all day, going from car to desk to sofa, then sleeping fitfully at night. A good way to tackle either scenario is to factor in time for good-quality rest.

What counts as rest? It's not so much falling asleep in the armchair, as doing something that takes you away from your norm. I always found if I was studying and losing concentration or starting to nod off, just getting up and relocating to a new environment helped. Or going for a brisk walk or jog. If you're stuck working from home all day, moving straight from your desk to the sofa is unlikely to be truly restful, but going outdoors into the natural world to take some 'active rest' might be. Likewise there are times when binge-watching *The Crown* will be just the mental rest you need from periods of intense concentration. Never feel guilty about taking time to rest – I certainly don't.

Rest means something different to each of us, and even to ourselves at different times. You could call it self-care or finding your 'flow state'. It might be a creative activity like painting, photography or craft. Maybe cooking or tending your houseplants helps you wind down. It could be working on your golf swing, washing your car, painting your nails. Or is it listening to music or a podcast, or reading a book? Sometimes you have to grab it while you can. Don't spend that bus or train journey answering work emails – plug in your earphones, close your eyes and daydream.

And that's a key point about emails, or texts or social media. I think we need to stop filling every minute of our downtime by reaching for our phones – that might be fun, but it's not restful. Sure, I like to do a quick Insta Story or TikTok post for you guys at the start of my daily walk. But after that my phone's away and I'm enjoying being in the moment and having some active rest.

If you're always exhausted without reasonable explanation, it's worth speaking to your GP. This can be a sign of nutritional deficiencies, particularly iron, B vitamins or vitamin D. It might also be a sign of stress and depression and could indicate other conditions – don't power on through, ask for some help.

TECH TIPS

Having said it's important to wind down without screens, there are some ways in which technology can help us sleep. First of all, most smartphones can be switched onto nighttime mode, which filters out the blue light with a warmer light source. There are also apps you can download to do this for phones and tablets, and even blue-light filtering glasses you can buy.

I like the sleep-tracking feature on my Fitbit because it tells me not just how long I slept, but also how many times I woke or was restless, and how long I spent in different sleep stages. I don't use it all the time, but it's good to check in now and again – and it's useful for spotting patterns, especially if you use it alongside a sleep diary (see page 174).

Trackers might not be useful for everyone though. I think if you're having real problems with insomnia, then having your device tell you in the morning that you didn't get much sleep could be highly annoying and might easily add to your anxiety levels.

You can also use a tracker or smartwatch, or your phone, to set a bedtime alarm – which is handy when you're trying to get into new habits or if you're someone who can easily while away hours scrolling or watching TV, only to suddenly notice it's midnight. Trackers and smartwatches that monitor your sleep can also vibrate gently to wake you during the lighter part of your sleep cycle, which is pretty nifty.

There are plenty of handy apps to help you fall asleep – everything from guided meditations and breathing exercises to celebrities reading soothing bedtime stories (or reading boring texts about things like economics in monotonous voices, I kid you not!). I'd only recommend these if you're someone who can be disciplined with your phone in the bedroom and resist quicky checking your emails afterwards.

Something I use myself is a sound-effects app – you can choose between things like soothing music, waves, a crackling fire, whale song and white noise, you name it. I like the sound of rainfall. It cancels out noise from the street and is particularly useful when I'm in hotels and unfamiliar sounds like the air conditioning are keeping me from falling into deep sleep.

KEEP A SLEEP DIARY

I think it's a really useful exercise to keep a sleep diary to check in with how you actually sleep, as opposed to how you might think you do. Be your own sleep detective and work out what the biggest issues are that you need to tackle. If you have a sleep-tracking device, you can use it to collect extra data and add that to the mix.

It's a bit like the food diary I suggest in Chapter 3. Not something you need to do forever, just for long enough to give you some personal insights. This is definitely something I'd ask a patient to do if they told me they weren't sleeping as well as they thought they could.

The first step is to ask yourself the following questions about last night's sleep:

1. **Where did you sleep? Did you sleep alone or with someone?**

2. **What time did you get into bed? What did you eat/drink/ do in the hours beforehand?**

3. **What did you wear? Did your bedroom feel comfortable? Why/why not?**

4. **How soon do you think you fell asleep?**

5. **Did you wake during the night? For how long? What did you do when you woke?**

6. **Did you wake naturally in the morning or with an alarm? What time was that and how did you feel?**

7. **How did you feel during the day?**

The next step is a task at bedtime. Keep a notepad and pen by your bed. Each night, before you get into bed, take five minutes to think about and write down your to-do list for the next day. Everything you need to remember for work, any bits of life laundry you're worried about forgetting. Think of it like downloading the busy bits of your brain, or powering them down, so you can stop the thoughts whirling round and let your mind rest properly.

You could use your phone to take voice or text notes, but I think there's something about the act of writing things down that really gets them out of your head. There was a study, published in the *Journal of Experimental Psychology*, that confirmed this works. Interestingly, it found writing down jobs still to do was more effective than recording tasks achieved.

SET AN ALARM

Set an alarm for bedtime, as well as one for the morning – set it a little earlier than you usually manage to hit the sack. Stick to both alarms.

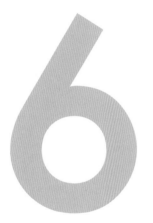 HUMAN BEINGS ARE SOCIAL ANIMALS. WE DO BETTER BOTH PHYSICALLY AND MENTALLY WHEN WE HAVE GOOD INTIMATE RELATIONSHIPS – AND GOOD FRIENDS – IN OUR LIVES.

SEX & RELATIONSHIPS

The ability to connect with others is an essential part of what it is to be human. Finding such connections – whether through platonic friendships or sexual relations – is fundamental to maintaining our physical and mental health. Bottom line: good relationships make us feel better, stimulate us mentally and might actually help us live longer.

But bonding with other people can be tricky, and making and maintaining relationships takes effort and – in some cases – a lot of patience. Increasingly in our fragmented world, many of our relationships are formed without meeting face-to-face. The use of technology to assist with making even the most intimate of connections with others has completely changed the landscape.

The number of dating apps seems to increase on a monthly basis and, as they become more and more refined, so too does the requirement to understand how to use them effectively and, more importantly, safely. The path to a long-term, stable relationship – if indeed that's what you're looking for – can be a rocky one. Not only do we have to navigate the minefield that is modern dating, but we all bring our own baggage and sometimes that can cause problems.

So whether you're looking for Mr or Miss Right or Mr or Miss Right Now, from a medical perspective, I want to ensure people pursue their relationship goals as healthily as possible, and that means mental health as well as physical health.

THE ADVANTAGES
OF BEING TOGETHER

Much research has been carried out investigating the benefits of a good relationship on our wellbeing. Warm, stable relationships can help keep us physically and mentally healthy and may even add a few years to our lives. Statistics show married people have lower death rates than those who are divorced, widowed or never married. Single people with heart disease are 52 per cent more likely to have a heart attack or die from another cardiovascular event than those who have tied the knot. And should your health decline in old age, a good relationship means you may cope better with any ailments you might experience.

Supportive relationships may protect your brain health too. People with a partner they can rely on stay mentally sharp for longer, whereas those in less secure relationships are more likely to experience early memory decline.

Before you all rush out and propose to the first person you see, it's the *quality* of the relationship that counts. Research found that midlife women in happy, long-term partnerships are at lower risk of cardiovascular issues than those in less satisfying relationships.

But it's not just about meaningful intimate relationships – your broader social network is important too. Social isolation is bad news for your brain – it's been found to be a strong predictor of a greater decrease in memory after middle age – but the health benefits of a good friendship are manifold.

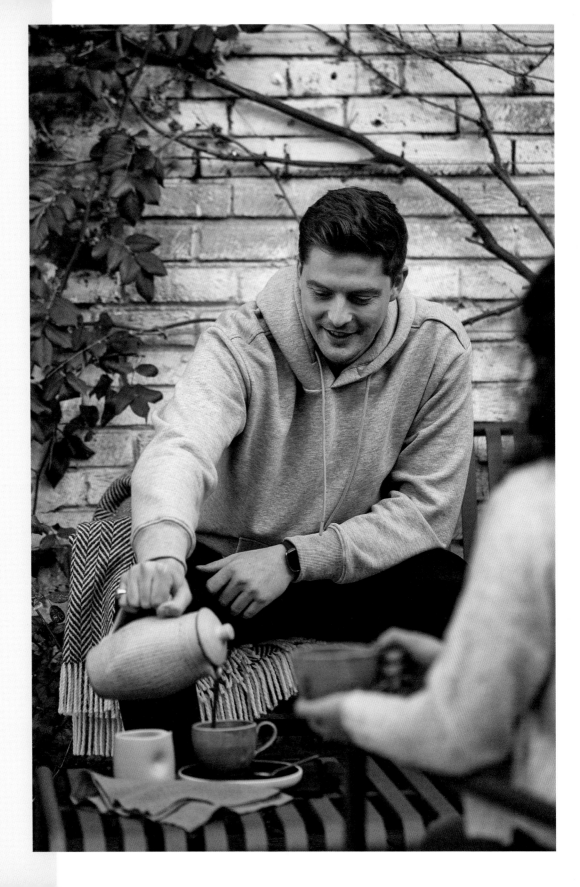

HUMAN BEINGS AREN'T DESIGNED TO LIVE IN ISOLATION – WE ARE SOCIAL ANIMALS.

ISOLATION

Having strong social ties could make as much of a difference to your health as quitting smoking, whereas loneliness is linked more generally with poorer survival, one landmark review of multiple studies found. So why is this? Well, human beings are social animals by nature and in modern Western society we're leading increasingly isolated lives, moving far away from family to study and work, settling down and having children later on in life, or not at all. There are higher numbers of single households than ever before. This isn't the way we're designed to live, so it's perhaps not surprising that studies show ten per cent of people in the UK describe themselves as often feeling lonely, and a third think they have a close relative or friend who's lonely.

Living an isolated life can step up the stress factor. And the stress connection is probably part of the reason a good relationship is protective. Some research has found loneliness triggers inflammation in the body, which is known to be connected to poor cardiovascular health. Scientists think loneliness can actually change the way the inflammatory system responds to stress.

Being in a relationship can therefore keep down the levels of harmful stress hormones in your body, which can be damaging in many different ways, including to the arteries, gut health and the immune system. It may also trigger the release of stress-busting chemicals. When you're in a challenging situation, even thinking about your partner can help regulate the physiological response to stress and keep blood pressure down. A partner may also play a role in encouraging you to look after your health.

It's not just companionship that's good for us; human beings have evolved to respond to physical intimacy. We're basically hard-wired for hugs. Children who aren't touched and hugged in infancy can have developmental problems. From MRI scans on adults, touch has been shown to result in lowered heart rate, blood pressure and cortisol, and rises in the feel-good chemicals serotonin and oxytocin. The result? Greater attentiveness, improved mood, an immune boost and lower pain perception.

LONELINESS

Two-thirds of 16–24 year olds feel lonely at least some of the time, and one in three in this age group feel lonely most of the time

43 per cent of people living together feel lonely

LGBTQA+ people are more likely to feel lonely than straight people (58 per cent vs 43 per cent)

Being lonely raises your risk of premature death by 26 per cent. That's similar to the risk of smoking 15 cigarettes a day, and is actually a greater risk than obesity and inactivity

If you are feeling lonely and have no one close to talk to, you can call Samaritans any time and speak to one of their trained counsellors (see Resources, page 233).

LOOKING FOR LOVE

You'd think that if I was going to find love anywhere, it would be on *Love Island*, right? Well, as most people know, that wasn't the case – I'm kind of hoping I can pick up some tips from this section myself!

I think it's fair to say that I was a bit of an outlier on *Love Island*. I was aware I wasn't quite the typical male contestant, but it didn't worry me. I was comfortable being different and being myself. I may not have found my perfect match, but I made some great friends on the programme, which goes to show you can find common ground even with people who, on the surface, are your complete opposite.

One thing *Love Island* did give me was an insight into certain ingrained attitudes that shouldn't really exist in the 21st century. For example, I think everyone should be able to speak openly about sexual relationships; in fact it should be encouraged. So many sexual health problems stem from ignorance or embarrassment. It seemed to me though, that while it was OK for the male contestants to talk about their sexual history openly and without criticism or scorn, the female contestants were referred to by their male counterparts in terms I'm not even going to repeat here. It's really not on – it's high time we ditched such archaic attitudes and realized that everyone, whatever their orientation, should be allowed to talk about sex and their experiences without fear of being labelled one thing or another.

This is particularly important in the current dating landscape. If you're single and looking for love – or something more short term – dating apps are the norm. Around 7.6 million people in the UK are estimated to use dating apps or sites. This doesn't, of course, rule out meeting IRL – but if you don't date digitally, then you'll be narrowing your field considerably.

SWIPING RIGHT OR WRONG?

Whether you're a newbie, an old hand or someone getting back into dating, it's always good to set some ground rules when using apps. Most of the tech companies have a duty of care to their customers, but that may only apply to the region the app is produced in. The good news is that the UK leads the way when it comes to accountability for online and tech platforms. However, it's better to be safe than sorry, so here are some things to bear in mind.

SAFETY FIRST

Don't go off-app

When you're first communicating, don't give away any personal details, including your surname, email address or phone number. Keep it on the app. Some experts suggest setting up a new email account specifically to link to your dating profile.

Trust your gut

Trust your intuition. If something doesn't feel right, pay attention to that. In the same vein, be on the alert for fake profiles. Be suspicious if someone:

asks you lots of questions, but doesn't tell you anything about themselves

has professional-looking photos showing someone with improbable good looks

is over-enthusiastic, gushing and seems to fall in love very quickly

uses poor language or grammar, particularly if they claim to be highly educated

gives you a sob story early on

says they're in the military or the medical profession – catfishers often pretend to have trustworthy jobs.

Never give anyone money

Do not hand over credit card details or agree to lend any money – even if the person you're communicating with seems convincing.

Meet up safely

If you meet someone for a date, tell a person you trust where you're going and keep in touch with them while you're out. Arrange to meet in a public place. Don't leave your drink unattended, avoid getting drunk and if you don't feel comfortable, make an excuse and leave.

SUCCESSFUL DATING

Safety aside, here are some tips for upping your chances.

DON'T...

...get into endless messaging

You want to find out a bit about someone before you meet – but weeks of messaging that doesn't lead to a date (unless there's a good reason, like lockdown) may be a waste of time. At least try to have a video chat to give you more of an idea whether there's a spark.

...take things personally

This is a tough one. It can be difficult when you meet someone you like and they end up ghosting you. But it's actually very unlikely to be anything to do with you. Remind yourself you don't really know them – you have no idea if they're very damaged from their relationship history, have personal or family issues that might be stopping them getting involved at the moment, or are still getting over an ex.

...cyberstalk a love interest

It's easy enough to find out things on social media once you've been on a date or two, but try to resist doing too much of this. It's better to get to know the real person, not a social media version of them.

DO...

...keep a first date short and simple

An elaborate date may seem romantic, but if you're not interested in the person when you meet, it may be a bit painful. Start with a simple coffee date or walk – if you're into them, you can plan something else for next time.

...be clear

Women in particular may be subjected to lots of well-meaning advice to play it cool and wait for the man to chase – but that's often unproductive in modern dating. If you're looking for a relationship, say so – it's less likely you'll connect with people who will waste your time. And if you'd like to meet up with someone, just ask. Equally, if you meet someone who seems enthusiastic about you, but you're not so sure, don't string them along to be polite.

...give someone a chance

If you think you like a match, but aren't 100 per cent sure, it's worth giving them a shot – there may be chemistry in real life. Similarly, if only minor sparks fly on a first date, it's usually a good idea to try a second and maybe a third, to see if things become more exciting. That said, you probably know when something isn't happening for you, so don't force it.

MOST POPULAR DATING APPS

BUMBLE

Who's it for?
Straight and same-sex couples.

The USP
Women make the first move in straight dating. For same-sex couples, either can make contact first.

How does it work?
When you match with someone, you have 24 hours to send a message, otherwise they disappear from your matches.

Good if...you're a woman fed up with receiving loads of unsolicited messages on other apps. This one puts you in the driver's seat. And it bypasses the old cliché that the man should make the first move.

But...you have to be quick, as that 24-hour ticking clock can mean you miss out.

TINDER

Who's it for?
Anyone, whatever your gender or sexual orientation, whether you're looking for long-term love, a casual hook-up. Tinder arguably normalized meeting a partner on an app.

The USP
The numbers and simplicity. It has a load of singles to match with, so you're likely to find plenty in your area.

How does it work?
Swipe right on someone you like the look of – if they've done the same, you're a match and can then send each other messages.

Good if...you want the process to be simple. Tinder can link with a Facebook profile for extra details and photos, so it's easy to get a good look and get swiping.

But...its upside can also be a disadvantage – the high numbers and the ease of swiping right can mean loads of matches with people you're not that into, which can be overwhelming.

GRINDR

Who's it for?
Gay men.

The USP
The classic gay dating app – you're shown a grid of available men in your area for chatting, dating or hook-ups.

How does it work?
Simple – upload your profile and you can swap pictures, chat and meet up if you want to.

Good if...you're looking for a big choice of guys very nearby.

But...the numbers can be a bit overwhelming. And you're likely to come across people you know, which may or may not be a problem for you.

HINGE

Who's it for?
Everyone.

The USP
You can use this app in a slightly more discerning way. Hinge lets you set tight preferences, including politics and family plans, and limits you to liking ten profiles if you're using it for free (you can pay and upgrade to like more).

How does it work?
In a similar way to other apps, but there are lots of preference options. And you can notify a match if you're ready for a video chat.

Good if...you're serious about finding a partner. There are no guarantees, of course, but the preferences help you weed out those who just don't share your outlook.

But...you're likely to have fewer matches, even though it's attracted many singles.

BADOO

Who's it for?
Everyone.

The USP
It's huge! It has over 380 million customers worldwide.

How does it work?
The emphasis isn't just on dating – it's location-based and you can say whether you want to make new friends or just find someone to hang out with in a city you're visiting.

Good if...you're concerned about safety, as Badoo has some tight security features. For example, if you're a woman fed up with 'dick pics', Badoo has a feature called Private Detective that detects these and alerts you to them, so you can choose whether or not you want to view.

But...you have to pay for a lot for the more advanced features.

COFFEE MEETS BAGEL

Who's it for?
Everyone, but especially those serious about finding a relationship.

The USP
Quality not quantity.

How does it work?
Instead of being given a raft of matches, you'll be presented with one each day based on your hobbies and preferences.

Good if...you don't have the time or energy to swipe through endless faces.

But...unless you get lucky, it could take longer to meet someone this way.

THE LEAGUE

Who's it for?
Everyone, in terms of gender and sexual orientation, but slanted at busy professionals.

The USP
This is more akin to virtual speed dating than standard dating apps.

How does it work?
Your social media accounts are 'vetted' before you're allowed to join, and then you're matched with 'prospects'. Two evenings a week, you get the chance to swipe through live video feeds of people who live near you who are on the app.

Good if...you want a change from the other apps – and users report finding the process fun.

But...you may not enjoy the cliquey feeling of having your social media accounts vetted.

TSER

Who's it for?
Trans and non-binary people.

The USP
It gives trans, gender-fluid and non-binary people a safe space to flirt and make friends.

How does it work?
In a similar way to standard apps – it has functions resembling those on Tinder, but you're likely to meet more like-minded types.

Good if...you've struggled with other apps and haven't always felt they're inclusive.

But...the pool of people may, inevitably, be a bit smaller.

**WHEN IT COMES TO LOVE, I BELIEVE
THINGS HAPPEN WHEN THEY'RE MEANT TO.**

MY EXPERIENCE: PLAYING THE LONG GAME

I've always taken a relaxed approach to dating – some might say too relaxed! Wanting to get into medicine from a young age and knowing what a commitment that would be, I accepted serious relationships would have to take a backseat. I did have a long-term girlfriend while studying at med school, but before I went on *Love Island* I'd been single for about four years. During that time I'd go on dates via apps and I did meet people who I clicked with, but none of the encounters led to anything, which was fine; dating apps offer an opportunity, not necessarily an end result.

Post-*Love Island* I was pretty wary of going back to the apps and didn't date very much for a while. The one long-term relationship I've had recently was with someone I met in a bar – quite old school! But dating via apps is *the* modern way – so many people meet online now and there have been lots of happy marriages and families as a result.

I'm not really dating at the moment, digitally or otherwise. I'm too busy for a start! I also believe things happen when they're meant to. If you search too hard, you'll either end up with the wrong person or you'll get frustrated. To be honest, the bar is set quite high for me. The strong relationship my parents have with each other has always been a big influence on my life. My mum and dad have been together for a long time, built a home and raised a family, and at some point down the line that's what I would like for myself. The kind of people I'm attracted to are usually very driven and passionate and believe in what they do. That's generally what I've always looked for and, if the right person comes along, then great.

But that's just me. The great thing about dating in the 21st century is that the technology can cater for all people and their different likes and desires, bringing people together based along those lines. Just remember, do be careful when using the apps and be safe when meeting your matches.

SHARED VALUES

One of the reasons couples like my parents are still together after so long could be that they have similar values. Values are what we feel is important in life – qualities we respect, beliefs we hold, principles we try to live by. Your values are intrinsic, something you feel deep within you. They're ideas about family, work, morality, spirituality, ethics. They're not about material things or external signs.

Research into successful marriages has shown that partnerships that last tend to be between people with the same values, which makes sense to me. Opposites might attract, but they might also make conflict more likely.

My point is, if you're looking for lasting love, don't get hung up on looks or salary bracket or having the same hobbies. Who really cares what car she drives, what films he likes or whether or not they're good at sport? It's more about whether you share the same sense of what's right and wrong; what's worth fighting for and what isn't.

POSITIVE PORN?

Technology has not only shaped the way we approach dating, it has also changed our attitudes towards sex. There is no bigger driver of these attitudinal changes than the availability of pornography. Once seen as something a little bit seedy and embarrassing, porn is now more accessible than ever before, available via multiple channels. So it's not surprising that surveys show 66 per cent of Britons have watched pornography at some point.

And the influence of that on our sex lives is very real. One in ten of those who look at porn rate it as being similar to real-life sex, with those who watch it more frequently the most likely to say this. Lots of porn-viewers try things they've seen – one in three men and one in four women says they've tried a porn-inspired move or two with their partner.

That may seem harmless enough, and in fact some research confirms that. For women, moderate use has been shown to have little negative effect on body image or sex-life satisfaction. However, when women are using porn for escapism from problems, it is more problematic. For men, the results are mixed. Frequent use of porn has been linked with more masturbation, less relationship satisfaction and more desire for porn-like sex – which may adversely affect a relationship. Excessive use of porn has been linked to erectile dysfunction, with some young men reporting they find it hard to become aroused by real-life sex with their partner.

That's not to say all porn use is bad. As with most things, it's about moderation. It can relieve stress, and if you're inexperienced or haven't met many people of your own sexual orientation, it can help to boost your confidence. It may also give you and your partner new ideas about things to try, as some research has found that watching porn improves sexual satisfaction by promoting variety.

The most important thing is to be honest with yourself about why you're using it and acknowledge if you're feeling hooked. Generally, if you're only watching it occasionally, if it's a part of your sex life rather than separate to it, and if you're not seeking out anything too extreme, you're probably using porn safely and even positively.

SEXUAL SCREENING

It sometimes appears that the responsibility for sexual health falls mainly to women and people with a cervix, so it's important to stress that it's essential for men to keep on top of their sexual health too. Maintaining an interesting and varied sex life can be great fun and also has health benefits in itself, but we have to remember we have a responsibility to our partners – whoever and however many they may be – to ensure we all stay healthy.

STIs

No one likes talking about STIs (sexually transmitted infections), but it's important we do. STIs are very common: in 2019 overall cases of STIs in England rose to nearly 470,000, a five per cent increase on the previous year. Young people (specifically those aged between 16 and 24) are most likely to be diagnosed with a common STI. Chlamydia is the one most frequently encountered, with genital warts the second, although that is on the way down, probably due to the HPV (human papilloma virus) vaccination programme.

Condoms are generally the best way to protect yourself, but they don't shield you against all STIs. Those passed on through skin contact – chiefly HPV and the herpes simplex virus (HSV) – can still be contracted even if you're using condoms, as they're not just transmitted through penetrative sex. In these cases, extra preventative measures need to be taken.

Vaccination against HPV is important – for MSM (men who have sex with men), girls and boys aged 12 to 13, and all those (up until their 25th birthday) who were eligible to have the vaccine but missed it when younger. The vaccine protects against the strains of HPV that cause cervical cancer, as well as genital warts. Those in higher risk groups – for example, MSM – are also advised to be vaccinated against hepatitis A and hepatitis B.

Regular testing for HIV (human immunodeficiency virus) and STIs is important for good sexual health – everyone should have an STI screen, including an HIV test, annually, and ideally every three months, if having sex without a condom with new partners, whether casual or longer term. It's also advised that everyone under 25 who is sexually active should be screened for chlamydia – either annually or when they have a new partner.

If you notice *any* unusual symptoms – discharge, lumps, bumps, pain on peeing or bleeding between periods – you should get them checked out.

KNOW YOUR ENEMY

CHLAMYDIA

The most common STI. Under-25s are the most affected. Typical symptoms for women include bleeding after sex, bleeding between periods and abdominal or pelvic pain, and for men, pain on urination, unusual discharge and pain and swelling in the testicles. But most people don't have symptoms. The long-term risk of chlamydia is pelvic inflammatory disease (PID) in women, which can start when the bacteria progress through the cervix into the pelvis and can cause inflammation and scarring in the fallopian tubes, which can lead to infertility and a raised risk of ectopic pregnancy.

What to do if you're worried

Go for a test – chlamydia can be treated very easily with a simple antibiotic. Recent sexual partners also need to be tested and treated, particularly as you can get reinfected.

How to prevent

Using male or female condoms helps keep you safe.

HPV

HPV is actually a family of over 100 viruses, and some of them are responsible for genital warts – small, fleshy growths that might crop up months after the initial infection and can recur. Other strains are linked with cervical cancer (these strains don't cause warts). Most of the time, though, HPV doesn't cause any problems and most people won't know they have it. Young people are now vaccinated against HPV strains 6 and 11, which cause warts, and 16 and 18, which cause cervical cancer (and may be linked with other cancers, like anal and oral, as a result of sexual behaviour too). The vaccine doesn't protect against other strains – but those other strains are also less likely to cause problems.

What to do if you're worried

You may need treatment if you have symptoms. But most people don't and what's key is to unstigmatize HPV – eight in ten of us will come into contact with it and the majority of people will clear it from their bodies naturally. But cervical screening is vital. If you come into contact with a high-risk HPV strain, over time it can lead to cell changes in the cervix – screening is designed to pick these up before they become cancerous.

How to prevent
While condoms can help prevent HPV, it's passed on easily through skin-to-skin contact. So it's not just connected to penetrative sex – it can be transmitted through any intimate contact.

GENITAL HERPES
Caused by the herpes simplex virus, this STI basically leads to cold sores down below. There are two strains, however – HSV-1 and HSV-2. HSV-1 usually causes cold sores around the mouth and affects 70 per cent of the population – it's often caught in childhood (when an adult with a cold sore kisses a child). HSV-2, meanwhile, only causes genital cold sores or blisters – it's less common, but more likely to recur. Like other viruses, HSV hangs about in your body after the initial infection. This doesn't necessarily mean you'll be battling flare-ups for life, but it might crop up from time to time, especially in the first two years after the initial infection, and often when you're run-down or experience other triggers, just as with cold sores.

What to do if you're worried
It can't be cured. But most people *don't* have flare-ups – the first outbreak is usually the most serious and, after that, any outbreaks tend to be milder, until they clear completely. For repeat outbreaks, your doctor may prescribe a medicine called acyclovir, which suppresses the virus and reduces symptoms. Although it's unsightly and uncomfortable, HSV doesn't usually have serious complications unless you have HIV, although pregnant women having an outbreak should seek treatment.

How to prevent
If you or a partner has active herpes, use protection whatever type of sex you're having, although it's best to avoid penetrative sex altogether. For oral sex with a vagina or anus, a dam (a small square of plastic) can be used to form a barrier between the mouth and genitals. Condoms don't offer full protection, but are still important, as genital herpes is caused by intimate skin-to-skin contact, through fingers and sex toys, for example. It can be transmitted even when there are no obvious sores, although this is less likely.

GONORRHOEA

The infection that used to be referred to as 'the clap'. It's been on the rise for some time and Public Health England figures show gonorrhoea cases jumped by 26 per cent between 2018 and 2019. It's now the second most common bacterial STI after chlamydia, although numbers are still relatively small in comparison. It can cause a thick yellow or green discharge, pain when peeing and, for women, bleeding between periods, although many have no symptoms. In fact, one in ten men and around half of women with gonorrhoea are symptomless. As with chlamydia, gonorrhoea can raise your risk of pelvic inflammatory disease and infertility.

What to do if you're worried

Gonorrhoea can currently be treated successfully with antibiotics – usually an injection followed by a tablet. But scientists are worried about a rise in cases of drug-resistant gonorrhoea, raising fears it may become untreatable. So prevention is key.

How to prevent

It's passed on in semen and vaginal fluids, so using a condom will keep you safe until you've been tested.

SYPHILIS

Much less common, but it is on the rise again. Symptoms can include small, painless sores around the genital area, though they can crop up in other places too, a blotchy rash on feet or hands, small wart-like skin growths and white patches in the mouth, as well as systemic symptoms like tiredness, headaches, joint pain and fever. If syphilis is left untreated for many years, it can eventually cause very serious health problems, as it can spread to the brain and other parts of the body. It's dangerous in pregnancy, so pregnant women are offered routine screening.

What to do if you're worried

If you think you've been exposed, it's important to be tested straight away, as early treatment is a must. It can be treated with antibiotic injections and you should avoid sex until treatment ends.

How to prevent

Condoms are the main way to prevent infection, although they don't offer complete protection, as syphilis can be passed on through any intimate contact, including the sharing of sex toys.

HIV

The virus that can lead to AIDS, HIV is most commonly spread through sex. Nowadays, it can usually be successfully managed so that most people with it don't develop AIDS and can live long and healthy lives. But it's still a serious long-term condition. HIV is still most common in MSM.

What to do if you're worried

Most people only have a mild illness at first. In fact, those infected usually have no symptoms until the virus starts to damage the immune system, often many years later, so you wouldn't know you were affected at all. If you suspect that you may be, however, you can be tested at a sexual health clinic, at your GP surgery or with a home-testing kit. If you're positive, you'll be offered long-term medication.

How to prevent

Male or female condoms are the best way to prevent HIV, and use a lubricant designed for sex as well – this helps prevent the small friction tears to the wall of the vagina that allow HIV to be passed on more easily.

It's important to remember that STIs don't always cause symptoms. It's perfectly possible to catch an STI from someone who appears healthy and may not even know they have an infection. So always get unusual symptoms checked out and maintain your annual check-ups.

WE HAVE A RESPONSIBILITY TO OUR PARTNERS TO ENSURE WE ALL STAY HEALTHY.

CERVICAL SCREENING

Anyone with a cervix registered with their GP is invited for cervical screening, otherwise known as a smear test, approximately six months before their 25th birthday. They are then invited every three to five years (depending on where you are in the UK) for repeat cervical screening.

The decision to start screening at the age of 25 is evidence based. Those under 30 who catch HPV usually clear it from their bodies naturally before it can do any harm. So if screening is started too young, it may lead to unnecessary treatment.

The way screening is done has changed recently. As we now know high-risk HPV causes cervical cancer, the sample is checked first for that. If high-risk HPV isn't found, no further action is needed and you'll be referred back to the routine screening programme. If it is found, a sample is checked for cervical cell changes. Depending on the grading of the changes, you'll either be referred for a colposcopy (a simple process used to look at the cervix, the lower part of the womb and the top of the vagina) or asked to come back in a year (the cells may well have returned to normal by then).

Being vaccinated against HPV greatly reduces the risk of cervical cancer. But it doesn't remove it completely. As I mentioned on page 192, the vaccine given on the NHS protects against high-risk HPV types 16 and 18, which are linked with the majority of cervical cancers. However, there are some other high-risk types of HPV not covered by the vaccine. So anyone who has been vaccinated should still be invited for and attend screening.

LETTING GO IS GOOD

As we can see, the people we surround ourselves with have a massive impact on our happiness and wellbeing, but as with many things in life, this is a two-way street. If we're in relationships – platonic or otherwise – that are no longer working, it's best for all involved that they come to an end. While that may seem an obvious statement to make when it comes to romantic relationships that have run their course, it may sound a little surprising applied to friendships. That's because we're so obsessed with the idea of BFF (best friends forever) that we find it hard to let go of people who we have drifted away from or who we no longer have anything in common with, or who even have a toxic influence over us.

This may sound a bit harsh, but I don't think people are always designed to be friends forever. You have your family and perhaps a core few people that you keep close, but for the most part, relationships come and go. Once you accept that some friendships reach a natural conclusion and that's perfectly OK, then it's easier to audit your friends regularly and see which ones are good for you and which ones aren't.

What's important is that, when you do let go of friends, you deal with it in a healthy way. While it's easy simply to unfollow old school friends on social media, it's not OK to ghost someone who you see on a regular basis. The best thing to do is take a break from the friendship and use the time to gather your thoughts. If the relationship has reached its natural end, then this may be enough for contact to stop naturally, but if you're committed to a regular social occasion with them, it's a good idea to let them know you're not going to be available for a while.

Get your thoughts down on paper, either in a journal entry or in a letter you don't intend to send. Externalizing how you feel can help you be clear about your goals and preferred outcome from the time apart. Once you have that in mind, you can either choose to speak to the person face-to-face to resolve any unacknowledged issues and put the friendship back on track or just sit tight, knowing you now have a valid reason to give should they question why you've not been in touch.

In most cases though, it will never come to this, as the lifecycle of a friendship is a totally natural thing. We all run different courses in our lives and sometimes it's good and healthy just to drift apart. While there's nothing to say you won't reconnect at later date, that too will happen naturally if it's meant to be.

THE RELATIONSHIP AUDIT

While tracking all the contact you have with people took a rather sinister turn during the pandemic, when it comes to assessing your relationships, this can be a helpful thing to do.

On social media all our relationships have a similar weight: a text message from your mum is on the same level as a round robin message from an old school friend you haven't seen in years. Obviously your mum is way more important, but in the moment when your phone buzzes and you get that dopamine hit, they're the same.

So by making an inventory of daily interactions, you'll be giving yourself the opportunity to look at who's really important to you in your life and makes you truly happy. Keep it simple; just make a note in your phone every time you interact with someone during the course of the day and how that interaction made you feel.

1. **Write down who you interacted with.**
2. **Was it a text, a call, Facebook message or face-to-face chat?**
3. **Was it work-related, personal, family or part of a service (a barista, for example)?**
4. **How long did it last?**
5. **How did it make you feel? Writing down one word will do: did you feel loved? Appreciated? Needed? Be honest.**
6. **If you're interacting with the same people at work or at home regularly, it may be easier to take a general view – you don't need multiple entries from your office receptionist, for example.**
7. **Try to keep it up for a week.**

After a week you'll have a good spread of interactions to work through, but let's focus on the positives – you want to pinpoint the relationships, and the ways they're conducted, that make you happy. Highlight the interactions that left you with positive feelings: was it getting caught up in a slightly dodgy WhatsApp group chat? No? Then leave that group, you don't need it. Were you happy to hear from a friend during work hours or did you feel anxious about being interrupted? The latter? Then put your phone on silent and call them back later. Did making small talk with the barista cheer you up? Then make a point to engage with people in shops or cafés in the future (plenty of research shows us how making a meaningful connection to a stranger makes us feel great).

Once you've assessed which relationships give you the most positivity, you'll know which to nurture. As for the others, maybe switch them to 'don't see posts' rather than 'unfriend'.

WHAT CAN YOU DO TODAY?

TELL SOMEONE

Take the time to tell someone special what they mean to you. Parent, partner or sibling, let them know that you're grateful to have them in your life. It doesn't have to be overly emotional or relate to any particular event, just a general thanks for being there. And, most importantly, don't ask or expect anything in return. You're giving a gift and affirming a relationship, whatever that may be.

7

SOME COMMON HEALTH ISSUES CAN BE TREATED AT HOME, BUT THERE ARE SOME CONDITIONS YOU SHOULD BOTHER YOUR GP ABOUT, AND SOME SYMPTOMS YOU SHOULD NOT IGNORE.

TAKING CONTROL OF YOUR HEALTH

The main purpose of this book is to give you the tools to take control of all aspects of your health, to try and ensure that you don't have to come and see health professionals like me. Later in this chapter, however, I'm going to turn that advice on its head and tell you about situations when I most definitely *want* you to contact your GP or, in extreme cases, go to A&E.

It's hard to know when to go and see a health professional. Some people go to their GP at the slightest sign of illness, while others put up with feeling discomfort, and in some cases pain, in order to avoid it. What I want is to encourage people to take an active part in their healthcare and to know when to treat an ailment at home, when to talk to a professional and when to call for an ambulance.

The advice I'm offering here is not diagnostic. Yes, I'm a doctor, but every patient is different and, without seeing people face-to-face, I can't make a complete assessment. So, while I hope to empower people when it comes to their health, please bear in mind that my comments are advisory and follow the guidelines of nhs.uk. The bottom line is, if you're worried, please seek help. It's better to overestimate a health issue, than underestimate it.

COMMON HEALTH ISSUES (AND HOW TO LOOK AFTER THEM AT HOME)

Let's start with seven health conditions that most of us are familiar with. Unless the symptoms are acute or persistent, you probably won't need to see a doctor for any of these, but they are troublesome nonetheless. In fact, this list includes the top three things people trouble GPs with unnecessarily. Can you guess which ones they are?

COMMON COLD

Everyone has had a cold at some point in their life. We're all familiar with a blocked or runny nose, sore throat, cough and sneezing. Colds can also cause slight headaches and muscles aches, which is why some people confuse having a cold with the flu (especially men!). There are marked differences though: a cold will generally appear gradually, while the flu comes on in a matter of hours and affects more than just your upper respiratory tract (nose and throat). A high temperature could also be a sign that you've got the flu. Both are viral infections, but flu symptoms are way more intense – you can carry on with your day-to-day business with a cold, but you'd be too exhausted to do anything if you have the flu.

There are lots of old wives' tales about the common cold, the main one being that you catch it by being out in inclement weather. If it's extremely cold and your core body temperature drops, then yes, your immune system could be compromised and you could be more susceptible to the virus. But for most people, if you're wrapped up warm and you're not hypothermic, going out in the cold will not give you a cold. In fact it's a virus you're more likely to pick up in warm indoor conditions.

So what to do if you find yourself with the snuffles? The main thing is to keep warm and stay hydrated, as any liquid you drink will help loosen the mucus in your nose and head. You can ease any aches and pains with painkillers and relieve a blocked nose with over-the-counter decongestant sprays and tablets, although when it comes to sore throats, a recent study found drinking warm water with honey and lemon is as effective as taking pre-prepared products.

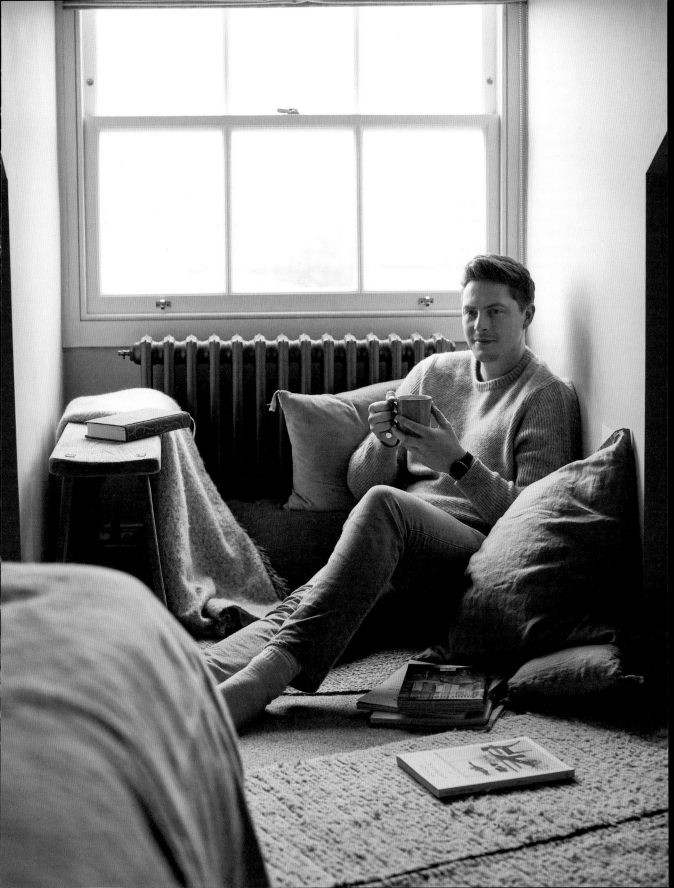

HANGOVER

There's always that moment when you first open your eyes the-morning-after-the-night-before and think you may have got away with it. But then you begin to notice the dry mouth, banging head and slight nausea that indicate that you have indeed overindulged and now it's time to pay the price.

A hangover is basically the result of overloading the body with acetaldehyde, a toxin that is the result of alcohol metabolism. It's thought to be more toxic than the alcohol itself and it causes the sickness and sweating associated with 'the morning after'. Your aching head is mostly the result of alcohol's diuretic properties, which dehydrate your entire body, including your brain. As for the guilt, well, you only have yourself to blame for that!

I'm sorry to say that there's no one-size-fits-all hangover cure. The best thing to do is to try and treat the discomfort as best you can. As the main cause of your ills is dehydration, it makes sense to rehydrate as soon as possible (you can even start this process before you go to bed). If your stomach is up to it, you can try soda water or isotonic drinks, and painkillers can help with the sore head.

Food-wise, it's best to avoid heavy meals that take a lot of digesting – so it's a no to the traditional fry-up – and drinking more alcohol, aka 'hair of the dog', is not recommended at all! Unfortunately, if you do the crime, you serve the time, so settle down on the sofa with a big jug of water and some mindless TV and just sit it out.

FOOD POISONING

Food poisoning is exactly what it says on the tin: something you have eaten has been contaminated with germs and has effectively poisoned you. The food may have been undercooked, not stored correctly or handled by somebody with dubious hygiene; and it's something that can affect any type of food. The results include nausea, vomiting, diarrhoea, stomach cramps, a high temperature and aches and pains. It's highly unpleasant and made more so if you got it from eating out.

The best thing to do is to try and stay hydrated with water or diluted sugary drinks – not fruit juice or anything fizzy, as they can exacerbate symptoms. Paracetamol can help if you're experiencing any headaches or other aches and pains, but the main thing is to stay at home, keep washing your hands and keep surfaces clean to avoid infecting anyone else.

SOFT-TISSUE INJURY

Getting crocked while exercising is the worst. Not only does an injury stop you doing something you enjoy, but if not treated correctly, it could cause long-term problems.

If you are unlucky enough to get injured, your first response should be to stop what you're doing immediately. Pain is your body's way of telling you something is wrong and continuing an activity when it hurts will only exacerbate the situation. In the case of a sprain or pulled muscle, follow the principle of RICE: rest, ice, compress and elevate. If you're in pain, then you can use painkillers such as paracetamol and ibuprofen. If symptoms do not improve after a few days, then speaking to your GP is advised.

But do trust your instinct if you suspect the injury is more severe. Breaks and dislocations, or any injury above the neck require a visit to your nearest A&E department. In instances like this, it really is better to be safe than sorry.

MY EXPERIENCE: SOFT-TISSUE INJURY

In 2014 I was lucky enough to go to Glastonbury. Unfortunately it was one of the festival's wet and windy years, so there was a lot of traipsing around muddy fields in Wellington boots. It was all part of the fun though. Well it was, until I turned my ankle over in a pothole on my way to see Metallica on the Pyramid Stage. I knew from the first flash of pain that the injury was quite bad, but I was at a festival and supposed to be having fun. So I just got on with it, probably with the help of some booze to numb the pain – not recommended!

I spent two days hobbling around before I got it X-rayed and of course it was broken; I had a lateral malleolus avulsion fracture on the outer bone of the ankle. Looking back, I knew something was up at the time and should definitely have gone to a medical tent. And that's my advice for you here: trust your instinct. Whether you're at a festival or on a sports field, if you're unsure as to what you've done to yourself, get it looked at by a medical professional. You would be surprised how even the most innocuous of falls can cause a break.

Oh, Metallica were great by the way.

INSECT BITES

Whether from a wasp, horsefly or mosquito, an insect bite is more an annoyance than an ailment. Common symptoms are red, swollen weals and itchiness, although in some instances the bites can be quite painful. In all cases though, the first thing to do is to remove anything left in the skin from the insect (or in the case of a tick, the insect itself) and clean the affected area thoroughly. Again you can apply the principle of RICE: rest, ice, compress and elevate. Try to avoid scratching the area, no matter how itchy it may be.

There are plenty of over-the-counter medications that can sooth any irritations, so speak to your pharmacist about those. Some people may have an allergic reaction to an insect bite, which can result in shortness of breath, dizziness or swelling, particularly of the face and mouth. If this occurs, seek medical help without delay – these can be signs of a severe reaction known as anaphylactic shock, which is very dangerous.

HEAT RASH

Heat rash is usually harmless, but can be uncomfortable and annoying. It's usually caused by excessive sweating, so is common during and after exercise. The condition is caused when the sweat glands on the skin are blocked, causing the sweat to leak into surrounding tissue, leading to irritation. The symptoms include small red spots, general redness and mild swelling, plus an itchiness known as prickly heat. In extreme cases, blisters can appear on the skin, which can lead to infection should they burst.

The best way to treat a heat rash is to apply something cold, such as a damp cloth or an ice pack wrapped in a tea towel, for no more than 20 minutes. Refrain from scratching the affected area or using any perfumed toiletries while the rash is present. Having a cool shower can help, as can changing into loose cotton clothing, so there's no excuse not to get out of your sweaty gym kit and have a wash after training!

If the conditions persist, seek advice from your pharmacist, who may recommend a calamine lotion or antihistamine tablets, but really the rash should clear up by itself after a few days.

BURNS AND SCALDS

While first-degree (minor) burns and scalds can be treated at home, I cannot stress enough that all burns have the potential to be very serious and, if there is any doubt, please visit a walk-in centre or A&E. The main reason for this is that the severity of burn is not always related to how painful it is – small burns can be very painful and larger ones not so much. Any burn larger than the injured person's hand needs to be looked at by a medical professional, whether it's painful or not. And for burns caused by chemicals or any electrical source, or that char the skin, treatment should be sought immediately.

Whether caused by a dry heat (burn) or something wet (scald) the first action is the same: get the affected area under cool or lukewarm water for 20 minutes. Do not use ice or an ice pack or any creams or lotions. Once cooled, remove any clothing or jewellery that's near the burned area and, if possible, cover the burn or scald with clingfilm. If particularly sore, painkillers can be used. And do stay hydrated.

If you follow the above advice for minor burns and scalds, the injured area should heal on its own within a week, as long as you keep it clean and avoid bursting any blisters.

It's a good idea to keep a small first-aid kit in an easily accessible place – keep it stocked with plasters, sterile gauze dressings, sticky tape, tweezers, scissors, alcohol-free cleansing wipes, thermometer, antiseptic cream, spray or cream to relieve insect bites, antihistamine cream or tablets, painkillers and an eye bath and eye wash.

HEALTH ISSUES YOU SHOULD BOTHER YOUR GP ABOUT

There are many reasons why people don't like going to see their GP. They may think their ailment is not important enough. Or they may be embarrassed. Or they may be a man (women are 66 per cent more likely to see their GP than men). Whatever the reason for your personal reluctance, if something is bothering you, then a visit to the GP is *always* worth it, if only for peace of mind.

In addition, people are often unaware that their GP can help them with issues that aren't immediately painful or serious. As I have experienced myself, the effects of conditions such as acne or fatigue can reach far beyond the ailment itself, and your GP is an important first port of call in getting you the treatment you need.

That's why I've put together this list of some of the conditions that you should absolutely go and talk to your GP about. You may be surprised how much they can help and what treatments are available to you.

ACNE

Being an acne sufferer myself (see box, page 209), I feel great sympathy for anyone with a serious case. Although a common skin condition that affects most people at some time in their life, it usually hits around puberty, when people are already having to deal with massive changes in their bodies as they develop. As a consequence, its effects are not only physical, but also mental, causing problems with self-esteem and confidence. That's why it's doubly important to seek help if you're a sufferer – your GP isn't there just for the ailments you can see.

Unfortunately for some there is no outright cure for acne, but the good news is it can be treated and controlled. There are lots of different options that you can talk through with your pharmacist, including several creams, lotions and gels available over the counter. If your case is persistent or more severe, if the acne appears on your chest and back for example, then your GP can prescribe topical or oral treatments as necessary.

There are also things you can do at home to help with acne. Constant washing can dry out your skin and make matters worse, so use a gentle cleanser to wash your skin twice a day and use a water-based moisturizer to keep your skin hydrated. It may help to avoid using make-up, but if you do, ensure you remove it completely before going to bed. If your hair is long, keep it clean and tied back to avoid it falling across your face.

If treatment is not effective in the time frame given by your GP, don't despair. Some may need expert advice and treatment from a dermatologist. Acne can take time to improve – there isn't a quick fix and persistence is the key. Don't give up.

ECZEMA

Eczema (or atopic dermatitis) is a catch–all term for a group of conditions that cause the skin to become dry, itchy and inflamed. It's extremely common and many people live with the condition without even knowing they have it. The dryness is a result of the skin being unable to retain moisture, and it can make the skin prone to reacting to triggers, causing soreness and inflammation. Triggers can include soaps and detergents, certain fabrics and

MY EXPERIENCE: ACNE

Acne can be a very cruel disease in many ways. People think you are unclean and dirty, and it can be incredibly stubborn to treat. I was plagued with acne throughout my late teens and I would go as far as to say that it crippled my confidence as a teenager. I once read a psychologist say that acne freezes the emotional development of a child at the age of its onset and I think there is some truth in that. I certainly became very self-conscious and often would not want to go to school because of it. I even battled with it at med school. In my first year as a doctor I had a bad outbreak and a patient commented, 'Are you sure you're a doctor? Surely you're too young with acne like that?' You can imagine what that did to my confidence.

I tried many different treatments, but at the time they were unsuccessful. This was mostly due to my impatient nature and inability to stick at taking the medications I was prescribed.

The good news is that, for the vast majority of people, acne *is* treatable and isn't something you have to put up with.

It's worth pointing out that one thing having acne has taught me is how to be comfortable in my own skin and, in a way, to be my own best friend. You can't allow what other people think to dictate your life decisions; there are enough critics out there already. No one is perfect – accept yourself as you are and be kind to yourself.

materials, hormonal changes (particularly in women) and previous allergies. Stress and the environment can also cause flare-ups.

There are several types of eczema, each one slightly different to the others, with its own specific treatment, so it's worth making an appointment with your GP, as they may want to refer you to a dermatologist for an assessment. It's important that you have a proper medical understanding of the condition to avoid any complications, such as bacterial or viral skin infections, as well as to know what triggers to avoid.

There's no definitive cure, but eczema is treatable with moisturizers and topical corticosteroids. Some products you can buy over the counter, but if the symptoms are longterm or particularly uncomfortable, your GP can prescribe stronger treatments.

As with acne, eczema can have a psychological effect on confidence and self-esteem, especially if experienced at a young age. Again, this is something your GP will be happy to talk to you about.

THRUSH

Being open about our intimate health is not something that many people feel comfortable with. But it's just as important a part of our overall wellbeing as eating well and staying fit. Take thrush for example: three out of four women will develop the infection in their lifetime and half of these will have repeat infections. And it doesn't just affect women either; men can be infected too, although it isn't as common.

Thrush is caused by a fungus called candida that is normally harmless. It can develop, however, if the balance of bacteria changes and tends to grow in warm, moist conditions. Thrush isn't classed as a sexually transmitted disease (STI), but can be triggered by intercourse.

Traditionally, thrush is identified by a white discharge from the genitals, as well as an itching and soreness in the area. However, thrush can also be asymptomatic, which means you may have the condition but you don't have symptoms.

While you can treat it yourself with over-the-counter medications, if you're experiencing symptoms for the first time, or you're under 16 or over 60, you need to see your GP or make an appointment at a sexual health clinic.

IRRITABLE BOWEL SYNDROME

It's estimated that 20 per cent of the population suffer from irritable bowel syndrome (IBS). That's a huge number of people experiencing some pretty debilitating symptoms, such as stomach cramps, bloating, diarrhoea and constipation. If you do suffer from IBS, it's something that is usually a lifelong problem, as unfortunately there's no hard and fast cure. Despite this, it can be successfully managed through diet and various medicines.

So if you do suffer from any of the symptoms above, or experience unexplained nausea, fatigue or incontinence, you should seek advice from your GP. Such digestive matters may be difficult to talk about, but it's essential to open up about them, if only to check that the symptoms aren't a sign of something more serious than IBS.

With any digestive issues, it pays to keep a food diary, so you can identify any triggers and eliminate those from your diet. It'll also be very useful when you have your initial consultation with your GP.

Many people who suffer from IBS feel embarrassed by it and can become withdrawn and avoid social situations. It's important to remember that you're not alone and that many people lead happy and fulfilled lives while managing the condition, but you *have* to reach out for help first.

Antibiotics can be life-savers for certain conditions, but we mustn't use them more than we absolutely have to or it can lead to antibiotic resistance. And remember that a course of antibiotics wipes out much of your good gut bacteria.

PREMENSTRUAL SYNDROME

If you consider that most women of reproductive age (that's puberty to menopause, about age 11 to 51) have a period each month, it's amazing it's not a more normal thing to talk about. I know from my friends, relatives and patients that so much of women's menstrual health is thought of as something you have to put up with. But that's just not the case.

Take premenstrual syndrome (PMS) – the symptoms you can get in the days leading up to your monthly bleed, caused by hormone fluctuations. Symptoms differ hugely, can be physical and emotional, and can vary in severity from month to month – making it sometimes hard to know what's PMS and what's a symptom of something else. It's worth keeping a symptom diary or using a period tracking app for that very reason. But if you suffer regularly from mood swings, feel tearful, anxious or angry, bloated or have tender breasts, suffer skin breakouts, fatigue, brain fog, headaches or changes to your appetite and libido in the two weeks before your period, chances are it's PMS. Lots of measures like regular exercise, relaxation and self-care, a healthy diet and sleep can help. But your GP can too. Certain medications, including different types of hormonal contraception, can make a huge difference, although you may have to experiment to find what's right for you. Don't be dismissive if you're offered anti-depressants, as in some cases a low dose is incredibly effective. Likewise, talking therapies can help you cope with symptoms.

Some symptoms can indicate a more extreme and debilitating form of PMS called premenstrual dysphoric disorder (PMDD), which you really shouldn't try to cope with alone. Likewise, if you have more physical symptoms, including severe cramps, bloating, or heavy or mid-cycle bleeding, your GP will want to know, in order to refer you to a gynaecologist (women's reproductive health specialist) and rule out more serious (but manageable) conditions, such as endometriosis, fibroids or some cancers, if need be.

LUMPS

Lumps on the body are completely normal and most people will experience them at some point. The majority of the growths that appear on the skin (skin tags) or small bumps under it (cysts) are not particularly problematic beyond being a bit annoying. However, should the lump get bigger or become painful, it's best to seek advice from your GP, as it may be an indication of an underlying condition.

When it comes to lumps in the neck, armpit or groin, or if you should find one in a breast or testicle, then it's imperative you speak to a medical professional. Don't panic; our minds often race towards the worst-case scenario, but there are a whole host of possible causes. The best thing to do though is to check your breasts and testicles for lumps regularly, at least on a monthly basis. There are many resources available online, including the Testicular Cancer Society and Breast Cancer UK. Lorraine's Change and Check campaign for breast cancer awareness is also a great source of information. The main takeaway here is, should you find anything untoward, see your GP immediately. The earlier these conditions are identified, the more likely a positive outcome.

FATIGUE

I'm not talking about feeling a bit tired after a late night – I mean a perpetual feeling of exhaustion that affects your ability to enjoy your life fully. A lot of people are reluctant to go to their GP with fatigue, thinking it not important enough to bother them with. The reality couldn't be further from the truth. Unexplained fatigue is common and could have far-reaching implications if not addressed.

The reasons for extreme and prolonged tiredness can be split into three categories: psychological, physical and lifestyle. Psychological causes are the most common and include stress, emotional shock, such as bereavement or a relationship break-up, depression and anxiety. All of these can lead to insomnia, which feeds into the experience of fatigue.

Physical causes are the result of specific health conditions, including folate deficiency, thyroid problems, anaemia and the side-effects of certain medications.

Lifestyle causes are probably the most insidious reason for fatigue. Modern living cultivates a 24-7 attitude to both work and socializing, so we try to cram too much into our days and indulge in behaviours that are not necessarily good for us as a result. Whether we consume too much caffeine or sugar to keep us going, eat badly on the run rather than sitting down to a healthy meal, or drink too much alcohol in the hope that it will help us unwind, these choices could be the reason *for* our fatigue rather than effective means to combat it.

Take an inventory of your lifestyle. Are you having too many late nights? Are you working long hours? Are you under any stress? Not only will this give your GP an idea of what's going on in your life and any underlying potential causes for the fatigue you're experiencing, it also offers you an opportunity to take stock of your lifestyle and see for yourself where the root of your fatigue might lie.

SIGNS AND SYMPTOMS YOU SHOULD NEVER IGNORE

So this is the section where I really have to use my stern doctor's voice – 'You must never ignore the following symptoms! Several can be dealt with by your GP, others by a visit to a walk-in centre and some will require immediate treatment, either at A&E or in an ambulance. All of them, however, are symptoms that can be indications of life-threatening conditions and they need to be treated by a health professional.' OK, stern doctor's voice bit over.

SEPSIS SYMPTOMS

Sepsis is a potentially life-threatening reaction to an infection that can lead to tissue damage, organ failure and even death. I have direct experience of the condition (see page 215) and I cannot overstate its seriousness. It happens when an infection you already have – such as pneumonia, infections of the abdomen and kidney, or even the flu – sends your immune system into overdrive, which causes inflammation throughout the body.

Despite its seriousness, it can be quite hard to spot as there are lots of possible symptoms. In my own experience, the main thing was an overwhelming feeling of something not being right and unexplained fatigue, but other symptoms include brain fog and slurred speech, pale, blue-grey or blotchy skin, and either difficulty in catching your breath or breathlessness. Some may also experience fevers.

The most important thing is to get treatment immediately; even if you're unsure whether your symptoms indicate sepsis, you should get to A&E straight away to avoid going into septic shock. Once there, you'll be assessed by the medical team and treated with medications such as antibiotics, if diagnosed with the condition. You may also need to be admitted to hospital for a period of time, until you have recovered.

EXCESSIVE THIRST

One of the main mantras espoused by health experts is the need to stay hydrated. NHS guidelines suggest we should be drinking six to eight glasses of fluid a day; that works out as just over one litre. It also pays to be aware of our thirst and respond to that, so if you want more than the recommended amount, then go for it. However, we need to remember that feeling constantly thirsty can also be an indication that something is not right. If feeling thirsty is accompanied by reduced peeing or dark yellow and strong-smelling pee, then you may be dehydrated and that will need to be treated.

MY EXPERIENCE: SEPSIS

About four years ago I nearly died of sepsis. I was working at University Hospital Lewisham. I cycled to work, as usual, to do my shift in A&E. But I had no energy for the ride and I arrived not feeling too good with a mild temperature. Maybe unwisely, I shrugged it off and got on with a busy day in resus. Once the day was over, I set off home on my bike, but struggled to cycle and basically collapsed when I got to my front door. I soon realized I was really unwell and was about to go to bed, but then, at the last minute, I changed my mind and decided to go to A&E. Looking back, it was that decision that saved my life.

By the time I got to St Thomas' Hospital in Westminster, I was mottled and grey with a really high heart rate, and I realized I was septic. The timeframe was 90 minutes from feeling unwell at home to being barely able to stand and struggling to speak in A&E. I must have seemed drunk to the receptionist, as I couldn't even write my name on the forms . A senior nurse walked past and saw how ill I was looking and rushed me through. Two resus units in one day – the irony wasn't lost on me!

I didn't need to go into intensive care, but I was on a ward for over a week and it took me six or seven weeks to recover fully. I never got to the bottom of why I became septic in the first place; all my respiratory tests were negative, but my blood markers were really deranged and my white cell count and inflammatory markers were very high.

I recovered though, and that was because I sought help at just the right moment. I'm convinced that, if I'd gone to bed, I probably would not have got up again. The main point I want you to take from my experience is that, despite the perception of it, sepsis doesn't just affect old people; it kills a lot of young people each year too, so be aware.

Excessive thirst can also be a symptom of high blood sugar (hyperglycaemia), which can be an indicator of diabetes. Excessive peeing when thirsty can be an early sign of diabetes too.

In these cases, going to see your GP or visiting a walk-in centre is strongly recommended. Even if it's something that's immediately treatable, such as dehydration, it's best to get a professional opinion.

CHANGES IN BOWEL HABITS

I get it, nobody wants to go to their GP and talk about what goes on in their bathroom. It can feel awkward and embarrassing to you, but I can tell you honestly, your GP will not be experiencing either of these things. They would much rather you go to them, should you be experiencing persistent or unexplained changes in your bowel habits, than stay home and suffer in silence. That's because any changes in your bowel habits could be an indicator of bowel cancer, the fourth most common cancer in the UK. Unexplained weight loss, mysterious fatigue, a pain or lump in your belly, bleeding from your bottom and blood in your poo are also symptoms.

The good thing is, bowel cancer is treatable and curable as long as it gets diagnosed early enough, which is why it's very important to overcome any embarrassment and seek advice immediately from your GP.

CHEST PAIN

The reasons for experiencing pain in the chest are many, and most of them have nothing to do with your heart. Saying that, a sudden, unexpected pain in the chest area can be extremely worrying, so it's better to seek medical advice, if only for peace of mind.

You'll find that, more often than not, the pain is related to heartburn, an infection, a sprain or strain (yes, you can pull the muscles in your chest), or an anxiety or panic attack. However, don't try a self-diagnosis; go to A&E as soon as you can.

There are rare cases when chest pain is exactly what you fear it is – a heart attack – and that requires immediate medical attention. If you experience a sudden chest pain that spreads to your arms, back, neck or jaw, or makes your chest feel tight or heavy, then you could be having a cardiac incident, particularly if the symptoms were preceded with feelings of nausea and a shortness of breath and sweating. In this instance, just call 999 immediately.

STROKE

There have been a lot of awareness campaigns around strokes in recent years and with good reason. A stroke is a serious life-threatening condition that can leave a sufferer with a range of psychological and physical issues, including paralysis, fatigue, memory and communication problems.

A stroke occurs when the blood supply to a part of the brain is cut off, so immediate treatment is essential. The symptoms of a stroke can best be remembered by the mnemonic FAST:

Face – the person's face may drop on one side so they're unable to move their mouth properly or one eye may droop.

Arms – the person may not be able to lift their arms and hold them due to weakness or numbness.

Speech – the person may not be able to talk or their speech may be garbled.

Time – if you see any of these signs, it's time to call 999.

I cannot stress enough how important the final point on that list is – the sooner a person receives treatment for a stroke, the more likely a successful recovery. It's also worth mentioning that strokes aren't confined to the older generation; the type of strokes can be different between the age groups, but one in four happens to younger people. Staying a healthy weight and maintaining a decent level of fitness are good ways to prevent against the risk of stroke throughout your life.

IRREGULAR HEART BEAT

I'm sure we've all experienced heart palpitations, those heartbeats that suddenly become more noticeable. There can be a lot of reasons for them: anxiety, lack of sleep, overdosing on caffeinated drinks, drinking too much alcohol, engaging in too much strenuous exercise and eating rich or spicy food. They may initially cause alarm, but in most cases they're harmless. However, they can sometimes be signifiers of an underlying health condition, such as heart disease or anaemia. As always, it's better to be safe than sorry. I recommend you visit your GP and get your heart palpitations checked out. If you're concerned, some smartwatches (including Fitbits) now have a PPG-based heart rhythm tool designed specifically to identify irregular heartbeats. That data can be shared with your GP, so they can monitor any issues you may have.

MENINGITIS SYMPTOMS

Meningitis is an infection of the protective membranes that surround the brain and the spinal cord. If untreated it can also lead to sepsis (see page 214). The condition kills a lot of people each year and, although it can affect anyone, it's most common in babies, young children, teenagers and young adults.

The symptoms include fever, stiff neck, vomiting, persistent headaches, drowsiness and photophobia (a sensitivity to bright lights). Other symptoms include a rash (that does not fade away when a glass is rolled over it) and seizures. If any of the above occur, you should go straight to A&E or, if a child is involved, call 999.

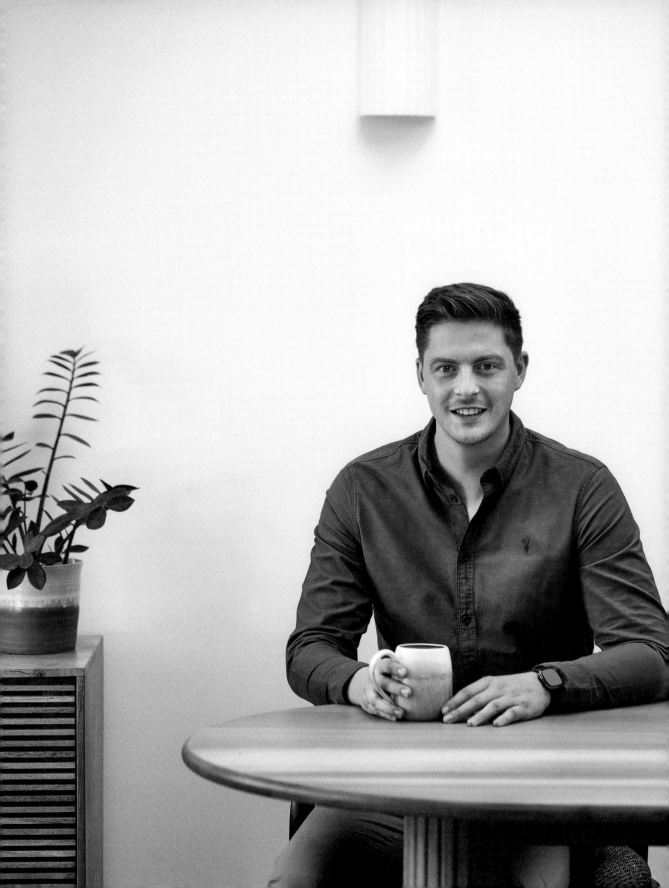

3
MAKE IT HAPPEN

7 THINGS I CAN DO TODAY, AND NOT PUT OFF UNTIL TOMORROW

At the end of every chapter, I suggest one small change you can try for a week. Even the tiniest one is an achievement, and a great starting point for lasting positive behaviour change. What can you do today that will make your life better tomorrow?

1 ....

....

2 ....

....

3 ....

....

4 ....

....

5 ....

....

6 ....

....

7 ....

....

HOW'S MY HEALTH DIARY LOOKING?

It's important to keep up to date with routine screenings and appointments, from dental check-ups to vaccinations. Make a note below of your last appointments and when your next ones are due.

NOTES:

PUTTING YOUR PURPOSE AT THE CENTRE OF YOUR LIFE

In chapter 1, I talk about how I found my purpose (see page 33). Make a list of your own talents, values, passions and areas of expertise, then think about how two or more of these areas could intersect – at home, at work or in your personal life.

TALENTS	VALUES	PASSIONS	EXPERTISE
What comes naturally to me	Principles and beliefs I live my life by	What makes me happy	My skills and/or qualifications

HOW AND WHERE COULD MY TALENTS, VALUES, PASSIONS AND EXPERTISE INTERSECT?

WHAT STRESSES ME OUT?

Our physical and mental health are closely linked. Keep a note of situations and events that make you stressed. They don't have to be bad things – good things happening in your life can be stressful, too. Identifying your triggers is the first step to dealing with stress.

NOTES:

ONE-WEEK FOOD DIARY

Keeping a food diary is a great way of getting a clear idea of what you consume and how it makes you feel. Include absolutely everything – it's easy to forget about snacks or drinks. Use the Notes section for any observations on your mood, hunger or digestion.

	MONDAY	TUESDAY	WEDNESDAY	
What did you eat and drink for breakfast?				
What time did you eat and where? What were you doing while eating?				
Any snacks/drinks?				
What time did you eat and where? What were you doing while eating?				
What did you eat and drink for lunch?				
What time did you eat and where? What were you doing while eating?				
Any snacks/drinks?				
What time did you eat and where? What were you doing while eating?				
What did you eat and drink for dinner?				
What time did you eat and where? What were you doing while eating?				
Any snacks/drinks?				
What time did you eat and where? What were you doing while eating?				
NOTES				

	THURSDAY	FRIDAY	SATURDAY	SUNDAY

MOVEMENT INVENTORY

We weren't designed to spend most of the day sitting down. Being active and exercising more is not just good for our physical health, but also our mental health. Keep a note of your movement levels for a week and then think about ways you could add more.

	WEEK 1	WEEK 2	WEEK 3	WEEK 4	WEEK 5	WEEK 6
MONDAY						
TUESDAY						
WEDNESDAY						
THURSDAY						
FRIDAY						
SATURDAY						
SUNDAY						

NOTES:

ONE-WEEK SLEEP DIARY

If I'm feeling more tired than usual during the day or more restless at night, I use a sleep diary to track the length and quality of my sleep. This is a really useful way of taking note of all the external factors that might be upsetting your sleep patterns, as well as acknowledging any changes to your usual bedtime routine and any worries preying on

	MONDAY	TUESDAY	WEDNESDAY	
What did you eat or drink up to two hours before bed?				
What were you doing just before bed?				
What time did you go to bed?				
Where did you sleep?				
What did you wear?				
Alone or with someone?				
Were you tired when you went to bed?				
Did you take a long time to fall asleep?				
Did you wake during the night?				
What time did you wake up in the morning?				
Did you wake naturally or with an alarm?				
Did you feel well rested?				
How were your energy levels during the day?				
NOTES				

your mind. Don't forget to keep going with the diary for a whole week, as that will give you a better understanding of your own sleep journey. Use the Notes section to record any events that might have affected your sleep – maybe a bad day at work or an emotional phone call – as well as noting what elements you could change to try to improve your rest.

	THURSDAY	FRIDAY	SATURDAY	SUNDAY

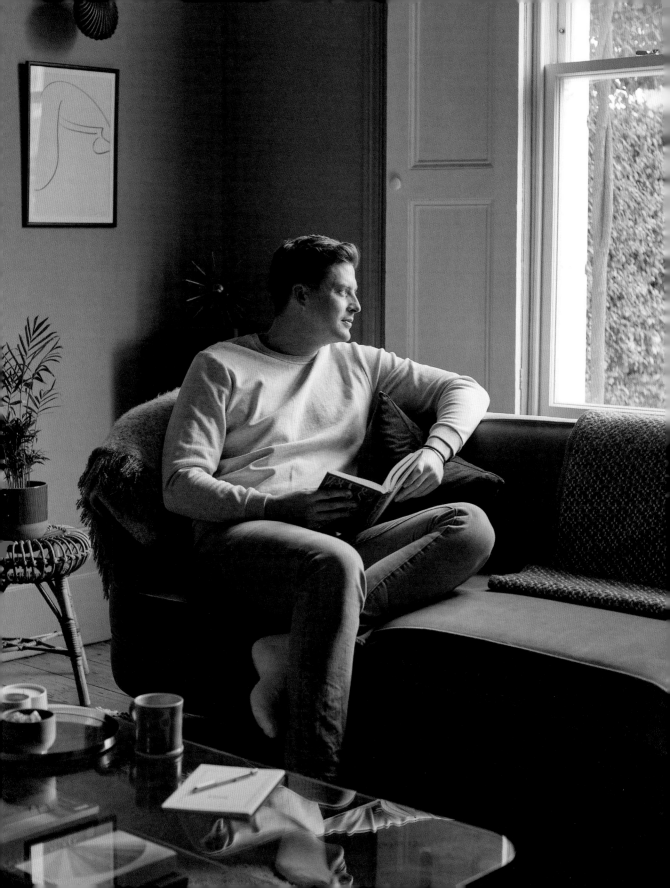

RESOURCES

GENERAL

nhs.uk

@dralexgeorge (Instagram)

@DrAlexGeorge (Twitter)

youtube.com/DrAlexGeorge

MENTAL HEALTH

samaritans.org

mind.org.uk

thecalmzone.net

NUTRITION

Eating disorders

nhs.uk/service-search/other-services/Eating-disorder-support/LocationSearch/341

beatingdisorders.org.uk

youngminds.org.uk/find-help/conditions/anorexia

youngminds.org.uk/find-help/conditions/bulimia

rethink.org/advice-and-information/about-mental-illness/learn-more-about-conditions/eating-disorders

mentalhealth-uk.org/help-and-information/conditions/eating-disorders

Healthy eating

bda.uk.com/food-health/food-facts.html

nutrition.org.uk

nhs.uk/live-well/eat-well

Weight management

nhs.uk/live-well/healthy-weight/calorie-checker

myfitnesspal.com

nutracheck.co.uk

Alcohol consumption

nhs.uk/oneyou/for-your-body/drink-less

nhs.uk/live-well/alcohol-support

drinkaware.co.uk

alcoholchange.org.uk

downyourdrink.org.uk

alcoholics-anonymous.org.uk

smartrecovery.org.uk

FITNESS & FLEXIBILITY

nhs.uk/live-well/healthy-weight/bmi-calculator

nhs.uk/live-well/exercise/get-running-with-couch-to-5k

parkrun.org.uk

goodgym.org

freeletics.com/en/training

RECHARGE

sleepdiplomat.com

Walker, M., *Why We Sleep,* London: Penguin, 2018

TAKING CONTROL OF YOUR HEALTH

pms.org.uk

mind.org.uk/information-support/types-of-mental-health-problems/premenstrual-dysphoric-disorder-pmdd

testicularcancersociety.org

breastcanceruk.org.uk

itv.com/lorraine/tags/change-and-check

ENDNOTES

A HEALTHY MIND

[1] Ziad K. Abdelnour

[2] www.mentalhealth.org.uk/publications/stress-are-we-coping

[3] link.springer.com/article/10.1007/s12160-015-9694-3

NUTRITION

[1] www.nutrition.org.uk/healthyliving/basics/exploring-nutrients

[2] www.nhs.uk/live-well/eat-well/the-eatwell-guide

[3] www.who.int/news-room/fact-sheets/detail/obesity-and-overweight

[4] www.alzheimers.org.uk/about-dementia/risk-factors-and-prevention/caffeine-and-dementia

[5] www.bhf.org.uk/informationsupport/heart-matters-magazine/nutrition/ask-the-expert/caffeine-and-atrial-fibrillation

[6] www.nature.com/articles/d41586-019-00398-1

[7] Jacka, F.N., O'Neil, A., Opie, R. et al., 'A randomised controlled trial of dietary improvement for adults with major depression (the 'SMILES' trial)', *BMC Medicine* 15, 23 (2017), bmcmedicine.biomedcentral.com/articles/10.1186/s12916-017-0791-y

[8] www.ncbi.nlm.nih.gov/pmc/articles/PMC3268700/

FITNESS & FLEXIBILITY

[1] www.nhs.uk/live-well/exercise/exercise-health-benefits

RECHARGE

[1] sleepcouncil.org.uk/wp-content/uploads/The-Great-British-Bedtime-Report-2017.pdf

[2] about.sainsburys.co.uk/about-us/live-well-for-less/living-well-index

[3] Dr David Lewis, 'Galaxy Stress Research', Mindlab International, Sussex University (2009)

SEX & RELATIONSHIPS

[1] health.harvard.edu/mental-health/can-relationships-boost-longevity-and-well-being

[2] cdc.gov/nchs/data/hestat/mortality/19-310689-Health-E-Stat-Mortality-H.pdf

[3] ahajournals.org/doi/full/10.1161/JAHA.117.005890

[4] health.harvard.edu/mental-health/can-relationships-boost-longevity-and-well-being

[5] Ibid.

[6] health.harvard.edu/newsletter_article/the-health-benefits-of-strong-relationships

[7] academic.oup.com/psychsocgerontology/article/75/2/367/5645554

[8] journals.plos.org/plosmedicine/article?id=10.1371/journal.pmed.1000316

[9] Ibid.

[10] sciencedaily.com/releases/2020/03/200305132136.htm

[11] sciencedaily.com/releases/2019/01/190122153854.htm

[12] sciencedirect.com/science/article/abs/pii/S0273229711000025

[13] relate.org.uk/about-us/media-centre/press-releases/2017/2/22/loneliness-rising-1-8-adults-have-no-close-friends

[14] relate.org.uk/policy-campaigns/our-campaigns/way-we-are-now-2016/friends

[15] rcn.org.uk/clinical-topics/public-health/inclusion-health-care/loneliness/recognising-loneliness

[16] yougov.co.uk/topics/relationships/articles-reports/2019/02/22/life-imitating-porn-many-brits-have-tried-somethin

[17] tandfonline.com/doi/abs/10.1080/10720162.2018.1532360?journalCode=usac20&

[18] onlinelibrary.wiley.com/doi/abs/10.1111/pere.12267

[19] nhs.uk/conditions/vaccinations/hpv-human-papillomavirus-vaccine/

[20] assets.publishing.service.gov.uk/government/uploads/system/uploads/attachment_data/file/914184/STI_NCSP_report_2019.pdf

[21] nhs.uk/conditions/chlamydia

[22] nhs.uk/conditions/human-papilloma-virus-hpv

[23] nhs.uk/conditions/genital-herpes

[24] nhs.uk/conditions/gonorrhea

[25] nhs.uk/conditions/syphilis

[26] nhs.uk/conditions/hiv-and-aids

[27] Petry K.U. et al., 'Benefits and Risks of Cervical Cancer Screening', *Oncology Research and Treatment*, Vol. 37, Supplement 3, 48–57 (2014), karger.com/Article/Fulltext/365059

[28] rcn.org.uk/professional-development/publications/rcn-hpv-cervical-screening-cervical-cancer-pub007960

INDEX

ACKNOWLEDGEMENTS

Having struggled with writing at school and university, which I later found out was due to dyslexia, I never dreamt that I would actually be the author of my very own book. My mother, Jane, used to make a point of telling me every night that I could 'achieve anything so long as you put your mind to it'. I think this constant positive reinforcement instilled in me a strong self-belief that I could overcome any obstacle in my way. What I later learned in life, particularly at university when struggling with my mental health, is that you do not need to do this alone.

Mum and Dad have always been there throughout the good, the bad and the ugly. Our sense of family, together with my brothers, Elliott and Llŷr, has got us through some of the most difficult of times. Although Llŷr is no longer with us, that family unit remains strong and I know that together we can overcome anything. This last year has been unimaginably difficult for us all, but in particular for my parents. I am so proud of them both and I hope that they will be able to find happiness and peace, despite everything. I know that Llŷr would want that. We have many adventures ahead and I am excited to do this together. I love you and thank you for everything.

As Live Well Every Day started to take shape, I remember how proud Llŷr was of me and what I was trying to achieve with this book. Like me he was passionate about health and felt that this book would give people the tools to improve their mental and physical wellbeing. Nothing will take away the pain I feel, waking up each morning and remembering that

he is no longer here. I have however found comfort in knowing how proud he was of me, which has helped immeasurably in getting through this time. Upon his passing, writing this book became one of the most important things I would ever do. I hope that you are proud of me, my boy, I miss you eternally.

Elliott, my outdoor adventurer of a brother, has always been the free spirit of the three of us. Particularly over the last few years, Elliott has taught me the importance of finding a balance in life. Striving for success and achieving your goals is important, but so is having 'care-free' time, living in the moment and not taking life too seriously. I am incredibly proud of you Elliott, you are living your dreams, working on fast jets in the RAF and kite surfing at the weekend. Keep living that dream. Thank you for always being there for me, throughout good times and bad. Be confident in who you are, you should give yourself much more credit than you do. I love you.

Alongside family we need our friends, they form anchors in our lives and are the source of laughter and joy as well as both comfort and strength. It is fair to say I have had a rollercoaster of a life so far and there is no way I could have stayed on this ride if it wasn't for the incredible network of people I call my friends. A huge thanks to my 'home friends' Adam, Mark, Steff, Craig, Daf and Sam – we have known each other our entire lives, every little flaw, and I wouldn't change a thing. I will never forget revising for my GCSEs and A-levels with you, Adam, camping out in my bedroom for exam season and pushing each other on. To be the best we could be.

At medical school I made the most incredible mates, we had so many amazing moments, my university memories I hold onto so dearly. We playfully named ourselves 'The Eagles', as we always joked about aiming high and living life to the absolute full, 'work hard, play hard' being the ethos. Thank you to each and every one of you for playing an integral part in making me who I am. To Chris, Vas, Ben, Morgan, Ella, Toby, Ryan, Joe, Jalal, Sarath, Dan, George, Charlie, Tom Yorke and Tom Blas, we continue striving to fly high. I must also pay tribute to Freya Barlow, a close friend of ours, who we lost far too soon. Freya, before you passed you told me to say yes and grasp every opportunity you could. I hope you are proud, we miss you!

Immediate family and friends aside, there are those people you meet in life, often in the most unlikely of circumstances or situations, who become integral to your journey. Many of these people I am now lucky enough to call my close friends.

There are lots of people who helped make this dream come true and were instrumental in bringing it to life. It wouldn't have happened without the belief and support of my incredible team at The Found Agency. I remember meeting my manager Harry Grenville as if it were yesterday. We instantly connected and shared an understanding of what it was we wanted to achieve. Harry, you have been a rock throughout the good times and the bad. This book would never have happened (and I mean this one million per cent) without the calming and assured guidance of Carly Cook, whose vast knowledge of publishing and

years of experience is matched only by her sense of loyalty and relentlessness to achieve our mission. I am hugely grateful for the ongoing guidance and support of Alice Russell and Francesca Zampi; I know there is so much more for us all to achieve as a team and I am excited for the future. I would also like to mention Lucy Smart and Sarah Foster, who I worked with before joining The Found: you have always cared deeply about my journey and I am proud to call you my friends.

To the wonderful Octopus team – Kate Adams, Jaz Bahra, Alex Stetter, Allison Gonsalves, Caroline Brown, Matthew Grindon and Stephanie Jackson – thank you for your support and guidance and believing in me and my vision for the book. We have created something we are all proud of and that I hope will do so much good. Thank you for being such a great publishing partner.

To my editors Hannah and Wesley – thank you for helping me put my thoughts, feelings and knowledge into words and helping to craft a book that I hope will help so many. Your wisdom and commitment have been invaluable. I have loved every second and am so appreciative of your help in bringing my thoughts to life.

I would also like to acknowledge a few of many important influences in my life from my years at school right through to my days working in Lewisham University Hospital. Thank you to Mr Martyn Harries at Tre-Gib Secondary for helping me believe in myself, to Professor Julie Thacker at Peninsula Medical

School, who inspired me so much and made me want to be the best doctor I could be.

Where would I be without the incredible team I call family at Lewisham University Hospital? I owe so much to these people. You have kept me grounded and humble throughout, always making me feel a sense of belonging. I have to mention Dr Anna Colclough, who essentially forced me to go on Love Island. Also a special thanks to Dr Nigel Harrison, who in my moments of despair following Llyr's passing shared a piece of advice with the that I will carry with me for the rest of my life. Life throws us into the deep end at times; however, with the help of family and friends we overcome even the most seemingly insurmountable challenges. Love and thanks to everyone at Lewisham Hospital, you will always have special place in my heart.

And my final thank you is to you, my supporters, my readers, who walk with me through every stage of this journey and who are my biggest champions. We have built a community to be proud of, a place where we lift and care for each other. Your support means the world to me. I couldn't do any of it without you and I never take it for granted. Thank you.

PICTURE CREDITS

Back cover background image: Woravit Worapani/Dreamstime.com

Additional picture credits: iStock Pra-chid 23; undefined undefined 160. living4media House of Pictures/Janmaat, Jeltje 41. Noun Project Heart by i cons 19. Shutterstock ITV 49, 70.